I0570609

THE ATHLETE'S FIX

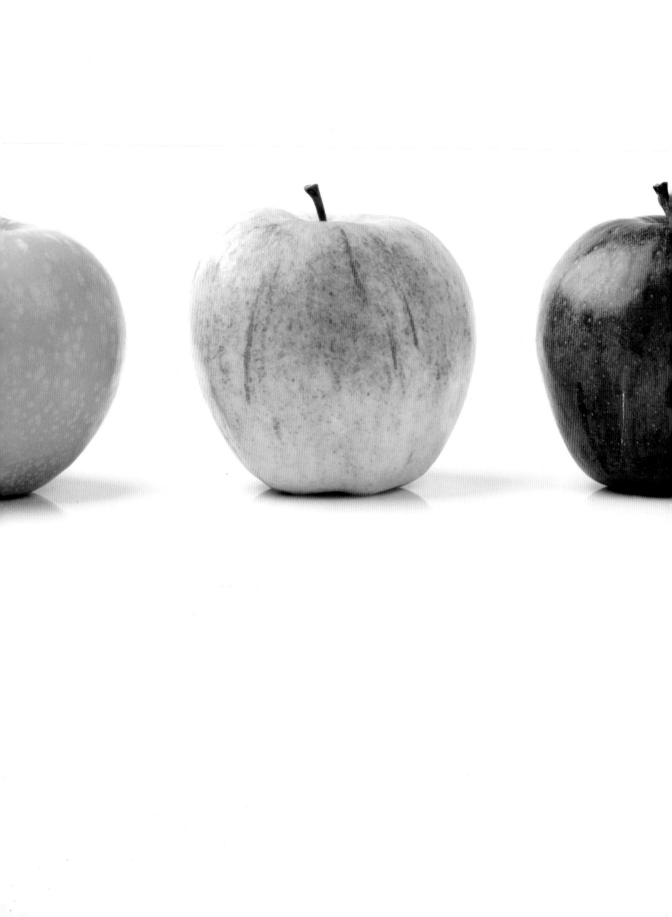

THE ATHLETE'S FIX

A PROGRAM FOR FINDING YOUR BEST FOODS
FOR PERFORMANCE & HEALTH

PIP TAYLOR

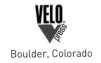

Boulder, Colorado

Copyright © 2015 by Pip Taylor

All rights reserved. Printed in the United States of America.

No part of this book may be reproduced, stored in a retrieval system, or transmitted, in any form or by any means, electronic or photocopy or otherwise, without the prior written permission of the publisher except in the case of brief quotations within critical articles and reviews.

▼velopress®

3002 Sterling Circle, Suite 100
Boulder, Colorado 80301-2338 USA
(303) 440-0601 · Fax (303) 444-6788 · E-mail velopress@competitorgroup.com

Distributed in the United States and Canada by Ingram Publisher Services

Library of Congress Cataloging-in-Publication Data
Taylor, Pip.
  The athlete's fix : a program for finding your best foods for performance & health / Pip Taylor.
      pages cm
  Includes bibliographical references and index.
  ISBN 978-1-937715-33-5 (pbk. : alk. paper)
  1. Athlete—Nutrition. 2. Physical fitness—Nutritional aspects. 3. Food intolerance. I. Title.
  TX361.A8T39 2015
  613.7'11—dc23
                        2015009389

For information on purchasing VeloPress books, please call (800) 811-4210, ext. 2138,
or visit www.velopress.com.

This paper meets the requirements of ANSI/NISO Z39.48-1992 (Permanence of Paper).

Front cover design by Pete Garceau
Interior design by Vicki Hopewell
Front cover photographs © Getty Images/iStock
Back cover photograph by Paul Versluis
Food styling and location courtesy of Adrienne Lee
Photographs by Rebecca Stumpf, except for pages 115, 143, 151, and 153 by Peter Bagi,
  page ii © iStock/Thinkstock, and page 2 by Richard Nolan-Neylan, courtesy of Revvies Energy Strips Ltd.

15   16   17 / 10   9   8   7   6   5   4   3   2   1

CONTENTS

NO LONGER PROPERTY OF SEATTLE PUBLIC LIBRARY

RECIPES *for the base functional diet*

All of these recipes support a BASE FUNCTIONAL DIET,
meaning they contain no gluten, grains (except rice), soy,
legumes, dairy, sugar, additives, or preservatives.

INTRODUCTION

Throughout my career as a professional athlete, eating well has been key to my performance. My diet has always been composed of healthy foods, and for most of my life I have stuck to a healthy balance of the widely recommended low-fat foods, including grains, pasta, couscous, whole-grain bread, and tortillas, as well as lots of fruits and vegetables, fish, meats, and nuts. I ate very few processed or packaged foods, in part because I have always enjoyed cooking from scratch and shopping at farmers markets.

Despite my best efforts to maintain a healthy diet and compete professionally, several years ago I began experiencing problems. My fitness and preparation were as good as they had ever been, but I found myself not feeling as good come race day. I was experiencing bloating, greater water retention—giving me a heavy, puffy feeling—increased lethargy, and shortness of breath. There was no reasonable explanation, at least in my mind—my fitness, health, and mental preparation were good going into the races. Per sports nutrition recommendations, I did change up my healthy, clean diet in the days leading up to a race by eating less fiber and fat to reduce the potential for gastrointestinal issues. Instead, I ate more refined carbohydrates: sweets, breads, and sugared sports drinks.

Because the most acute problems were happening when I raced, I figured they might be related to the carbo-loading I was doing prior to race day—which was often heavy on gluten-containing breads or cereals. So I cut gluten out of my pre-race diet. Right away, I felt like I could breathe better on race day—it was somehow easier.

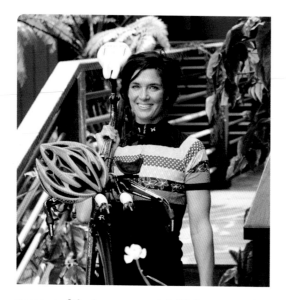

Because of the improvement, I didn't see a need to make additional changes to my daily diet; I simply focused on eliminating bread, pasta, and wheat-based cereals. I still ate some packaged foods with trace amounts of gluten, but I wasn't overly strict. In other words, I was confident I did not have celiac disease but understood that a low-gluten diet seemed to work better for me. As time went on, I continued to notice a difference, although it wasn't as pronounced as it had been at first. The difficult breathing episodes seemed to abate, but my on-again, off-again habits were bringing new issues to my attention. If racing was going to be my livelihood and profession, I knew I needed to figure out exactly which foods were leading to setbacks.

I began researching food intolerances and their effects on the body, eliminating specific foods in a more conscientious way, and taking note of the different impacts those dietary adjustments had on my body, mind, and athletic performance. This wasn't an entirely random process, as I drew on my scientific nutritional education and knowledge in combination with personal experience.

By strictly avoiding all inflammatory foods and my own identified "trigger foods," such as gluten and grains, and by reducing my reliance on carbohydrate-heavy foods, I found that my body weight was easier to maintain. The headaches I had endured for years lifted, along with the brain fog, which did wonders for my mood and encouraged me to continue to make better food choices. I focused more on proteins such as fish, poultry, and meats and included plenty of healthy natural fats along with an abundance of vegetables and fruits. The improvements were obvious. To my surprise, I didn't miss eating grains, and I found myself to be less hungry in general. I felt physically and mentally strong when I ate the right foods.

Looking back, I believe there were other signs of my food intolerances and sensitivities, starting with those headaches I had endured for years. I assumed everyone experienced a headache at some level from time to time, so unless the severity ramped up, headaches really didn't bother me. At one point they were so frequent, almost constant, that I couldn't remember not having one. Because I tend to hold tension in my neck and shoulders, tightness through these areas would cause my headaches to worsen. But even with massage, stretching, physical therapy, and strict attention to postural habits, the headaches persisted. I had my eyes checked, my hearing and balance checked; I even had some other scans and tests done just to make sure the headaches weren't the result of some other medical issue, but all the results came back showing nothing was wrong.

Iron deficiency was yet another issue that I dealt with from a young age. While I've never restricted meat, my iron levels have always been quite low, sometimes reduced to trace levels. Even with prescribed supplements, it was difficult for me to maintain acceptable levels of iron. Growing up, I was consistently training with an elite swimming squad, making national age squads and collecting state junior medals, and I competed in junior running competitions too, though I spent little time actually training for running. Despite lack of run volume, I suffered from multiple stress fractures, which were quickly attributed to the process of growing. As I met with success on the track, I took a more conscientiously focused approach to my training, but the stress fractures only increased. The problem persisted as I started competing in triathlon, despite no identifiable cause. I have always had access to extremely good doctors, but they had no satisfactory explanation for my stress fractures, iron deficiencies, or any of my other symptoms. When a fit and healthy person is facing ongoing problems that the medical world can't explain, it's time to take a hard look at diet.

For me, this exploratory journey became both personal and professional. Through formal study, including a master's degree in nutrition and dietetics, as well as credentials in sports nutrition and dietetics, research, and experience working with others, I have found that changes in diet can have profound effects on health as well as performance. I have also discovered that sometimes the results of dietary changes can't be confirmed through definitive tests. But the proof really lies in the individual's response, whether it is a significant change in body weight and composition, reduction or complete elimination of long-term troubling symptoms, or the results chalked up on competition day.

Athletes place great demands on their bodies, and over time training and racing can expose problems that compromise performance and health. Most athletes embrace a reasonably healthy diet to support their active lifestyle, but it's easy to stop short of finding the answers to all of our questions or resolving nagging issues, however obvious or inconsequential they might seem. Chances are good that there's some room for improvement in your own diet. Ask yourself the questions on the next page to determine if your diet is helping you perform at your highest level. What you eat may have a starring or supporting role in any one of these issues. Of course all of these questions also involve other factors, but diet undeniably contributes to these problems, and it's a factor that is in our power to control and change.

When it comes to nutrition, mixed messages and confusion often go hand in hand. It's funny that we have such a hard time knowing what exactly we should or shouldn't be eating, since it's something we all do multiple times a day. An athlete's confusion over food is no different. It's widely recognized that good nutrition is an integral part of any training program and essential for helping you perform at your best, but there seems to be a lack of understanding about just what makes a good athletic diet, in addition to what makes a healthy diet generally.

The fix for athletes—and for everyone else, for that matter—is to eat as wide a variety of beneficial foods as possible while avoiding or minimizing foods that have a negative impact on health, performance, or both. Too many diets aggressively eliminate foods as a one-size-fits-all solution to better health. It's common to experience positive

What are you **LOOKING TO FIX?**

○ Are you frustrated by unsuccessful attempts to lose weight?
○ Do you find yourself craving certain foods?
○ Do you suffer from headaches?
○ Does your skin break out in rashes, dry patches, or acne?
○ Are gastrointestinal (GI) issues a daily or common occurrence?
○ Do you struggle to add lean muscle and develop power and strength?
○ Do you feel as though your race performance is not meeting your expectations?
○ Does your training route have to take into account bathroom stops?
○ Do you suffer from GI distress during competition?
○ Do you feel as though your ability to recover from training is declining?
○ Are you missing workouts due to frequent illnesses and nagging injuries?
○ Do you struggle to make quick tactical decisions under pressure?
○ Despite being fit, do you sometimes find it hard to breathe?

results from changing up your diet in this way, though you will not know exactly why the change is working. You might benefit even more by reintroducing some of those restricted foods to maximize variety in your diet. I believe that there is little point in eliminating foods without reason. Food, like life, is to be enjoyed. By the same token, you want to ensure that the foods you do eat are positively adding to your ability to play, train, or race to your best ability while also supporting a long and healthy life. To identify the foods that could be to blame for the issues you face, you will need to take a more careful approach.

A key component to any healthy diet is being able to enjoy food. Far more than simply sustaining life, food is social, and it is meant to be enjoyed. Customs, traditions, and connectivity to others are all wrapped up in growing, preparing, and eating food. The extent to which we enjoy food and the rituals around it is also important to health. After all, you can't have a healthy body without a healthy mind. And there is no point in living a long, healthy life if it is not enjoyable too. Eating is something we need to do every day, multiple times throughout the day. I love food and I want to help you make your experience with food truly enjoyable, regardless of what food intolerances or sensitivities you bring to the table.

The Athlete's Fix is designed to help you become aware of your own food intolerances, be confident in making healthy food choices, and eat the foods that are optimal *for you*. Once you find your best diet, better health and performance are within reach.

Comparing *POPULAR DIETS* *to the* BASE FUNCTIONAL DIET

In their best form, all these diets emphasize real foods: lots of fruits and vegetables, good-quality protein sources, and healthy fats. There are differences, though, in the logic behind each diet, as well as its applications. The base functional diet I propose is focused on helping athletes achieve better health and performance by identifying their own best diet.

Paleo. Contrary to popular opinion, the Paleo Diet is not just meat-centric but includes many fruits and vegetables. Paleo advocates will find many familiar concepts (and foods) emphasized in the base functional diet: fruits and vegetables, proteins, nuts, and natural fats. Both diets avoid sugar, processed foods and additives, wheat and other grains, legumes, and dairy. The rationale and endpoints for the two diets, however, are different. The base functional diet is not concerned with history and what was or wasn't available to our ancestors, but rather focuses on the best foods available to us now, eliminating those that most likely contribute to symptoms, in other words, the most common allergens and sources of intolerances. The base functional diet eliminates foods to begin with, but then encourages reintroduction of whole foods including dairy, whole grains, and legumes

(prepared properly), according to an individual's tolerance for them. The base functional diet also includes rice and rice products, such as rice noodles and rice flour, as low-allergenic, well-tolerated foods that help provide energy and variety to the diet. Both diets have a strong focus on real foods.

Whole30. This program is similar to Paleo, but goes another step by not allowing any sweet foods such as honey or desserts made with Paleo-approved ingredients. The idea is to follow the program for 30 days in an effort to heal, change tastes, and break poor habits. There are similarities with the base functional diet, such as an emphasis on whole, real foods, but the goal of the base functional diet is to promote long-term health as well as to identify individual intolerances, with the potential of reintroducing foods. Non-Whole30

foods such as desserts and flour-based foods, including baked goods, are included in the base functional diet and are more practical for the needs of high-energy, generally healthy athletes.

Dukan. The Dukan Diet is primarily a high-protein, low-carb weight-loss diet that takes dieters through four different stages in which certain foods are allowed or restricted. Fat-free foods are encouraged, as well as non-caloric sweeteners and other packaged foods as long as they do not breach the set caloric and carbohydrate levels. A celebration food is also scheduled in. This diet is likely not suitable for high-intensity or endurance athletes, and the focus is more on weight loss rather than long-term health or individual intolerances. *Continued*

Comparing POPULAR DIETS *Continued*

Mediterranean. Like the base functional diet, the Mediterranean Diet emphasizes whole real foods. But whole grains and legumes are encouraged, and saturated fats (even natural ones) are discouraged. Fish, other seafood, and poultry are prioritized over red meats. The Mediterranean Diet has much to recommend it in terms of natural unprocessed foods, but no attention is paid to identification and elimination of individual intolerances.

Detox. Detox diets are usually followed for a short period of time and often consist of fruit and vegetable juices and little else, with the goal of fast weight loss. The human body is adept at detoxifying itself, provided that a healthy, nutritious diet is followed,so there is no evidence that a detox diet is needed. The base functional diet takes a long-term approach to health and is not just focused on weight loss or a quick fix, but rather on individual health and longevity.

Dash. The DASH (Dietary Approaches to Stop Hypertension [high blood pressure]) Diet also reduces processed and packaged foods, encouraging followers to increase consumption of fruits and vegetables as well as lean proteins, nuts, and whole grains. The DASH Diet has also helped people lose weight and increase health. Similar to the Mediterranean Diet, the DASH Diet does not allow for systematic identification of individual intolerances.

Vegetarian/vegan. These diets focus on plant foods, including whole grains, soy (a common allergen), and legumes, and animal products are avoided. Meeting some nutritional requirements can be challenging on a vegetarian diet, and for some athletes obtaining adequate energy can be problematic. It is also possible to follow a vegetarian diet and yet consume many processed foods. Both vegetarian diets and the base functional diet embrace plenty of whole real foods. For more details on the base functional diet for vegans and vegetarians, see page 47.

Raw food. This is another diet that emphasizes natural foods; however, a raw diet is restrictive by its very nature and difficult to follow, and it's harder for most athletes to obtain sufficient energy and nutrients to sustain activity. Some foods retain all their nutrients when eaten raw, but others are actually more nutritious when cooked. A healthy diet comprises both raw and cooked foods.

Traditional elimination. The elimination diet echoes some of the principles of the base functional diet in that the goal is to identify intolerances through a systematic approach. Unlike the base functional diet, though, little attention is paid to inflammatory foods such as sugar and processed foods. These foods are allowed as long as they don't include the stipulated ingredients.

Too many diets aggressively eliminate foods. It's common to experience short-term positive results from changing up your diet in this way, though you will not know exactly WHY THE CHANGE IS WORKING.

THE PROBLEM OF FOOD INTOLERANCE

Food acts as fuel for our bodies, whether for the busyness of everyday life or the heat of competition. But the role of food extends beyond function to define our social and cultural identity. Food is central to many of our strongest memories and adds richness to experiences and relationships. Food can also be medicinal, both nourishing and healing. Unfortunately, eating the wrong foods can be every bit as detrimental to your health as eating the right foods is beneficial. It's a fact that's lost on many people, either because they choose to ignore or find ways to deal with the problems brought on by their diets or because for the time being, their bodies are more resilient than others'. For the majority of people, diet adjustment is one of the easiest lifestyle changes you can make to maximize positive genetic predispositions and abilities.

Because sports place physical and mental strain on the body, a healthy diet is even more important for athletes. When your body is not trying to fight itself, for example by combating inflammation inflicted by what you are eating, it is only logical that you will recover better and experience more optimal performance. The right foods will improve recovery and resilience, whether you are an Ironman® triathlete training five to seven hours a day or a professional baseball player in the middle of a 162-game season. A healthy diet can also reduce or eliminate the gastrointestinal symptoms that threaten to sideline athletes and leave hard-fought goals in the gutter. In sports like gymnastics, diving, soccer, or football, focus and mental clarity play a huge role, and eating the foods that facilitate brain function can increase sharpness and decision making. Being mentally alert also factors into endurance sports, reducing the risk of injury due to a misplaced foot or a fall. In addition, finding your best foods will allow you to reach and maintain the ideal body composition for your particular sport, whether that is lean and light or muscular and powerful. Understanding how your body responds to and tolerates various foods and what your unique needs are sets you up for better performance and faster recovery, as well as physical and mental resilience.

WHERE THE PROBLEM STARTS

WHAT HAPPENS DURING DIGESTION

When you sit down to a plate of food or peruse a menu, you might think that you are about to feed your body with fuel for working muscles and energy for brain cells. It seems like a simple matter of providing the essential proteins and fats, vitamins and minerals to keep all your internal mechanisms happily ticking along. This neat yet overly simplistic account skips over some important truths and oversimplifies the body's process of digesting and processing food.

The gastrointestinal tract is a long tube that is the point of entry for the food we need for metabolism as well as the exit for waste. Throughout, the complex digestive system is constantly interacting with the body's other systems. This is an important concept to understand because when someone eats a food he or she cannot tolerate, reactions can occur anywhere in the body. Skin reactions, headaches, and trouble concentrating are all among potential symptoms of food intolerance. Just because you don't suffer from stomachaches and aren't constantly running for the closest toilet doesn't mean you have no food intolerances. In fact, it's very common to have zero stomach complaints and still have trouble with certain foods.

The gastrointestinal system is designed to digest and absorb proteins, carbohydrates, and fats as well as nutrients, trace mineral elements, and fluids from the food and drinks we consume. The semipermeable barrier that forms the gut wall is the real point where food enters the body. But it is also the major point of contact with the external environment, and as such plays a key role in the complex processes of the immune system. In fact, over 70 percent of the immune system is located within the gut.[1] Every day your GI tract is exposed to both beneficial nutrients and potential toxins such as bacteria and viruses. A healthy gut wall will selectively allow nutrients and other necessary substances to enter the body and block out unwanted and potentially dangerous molecules.

Think of the gut barrier as a brick wall, with the cells that line the gut serving as the bricks. The mortar in between the bricks forms tight junctions. Some substances such as nutrients are small enough to sneak through these junctions (that's a good thing). Under stress, the brick wall becomes unstable and the gaps between the bricks get bigger, increasing the permeability of the gut barrier to allow in substances that are usually too big to pass through the gut wall and into the body, which isn't such a good thing. This situation is often referred to as leaky gut.[2] Partially digested foods, bacteria, viruses, and other toxins can enter the bloodstream when you have a leaky gut. Once in the bloodstream, these particles are recognized as foreign invaders, causing the body to launch an inflammatory response. Ongoing or chronic inflammation can result in the presentation of many symptoms and lead to many serious health conditions.[3] By investigating your own food intolerances, you can identify contributors to a leaky gut and the inflammation and irritation that follow.

HOW HEALTHY IS YOUR GUT?

There is much more to the story. It's not just our response to the food we eat that factors into digestion and good health. Why? Because less than 10 percent of the cells in our body are our own. The rest, over 100 trillion cells, are comprised of bacteria, the majority of which reside in our large intestines.[4]

The bacteria in your gut make up a complex microcosm responsible for helping to digest your food, breaking down carbohydrates not digested in the upper gut, producing hormones and vital nutrients, including vitamins B and K, and playing a crucial role in your immune system. Carbohydrates fermented in the gut break down to

What are probiotics and prebiotics?

Probiotics are commonly referred to as the "good" bacteria—live microorganisms that can help establish or maintain a good microflora in your gut. Probiotic foods include kimchi, sauerkraut, and other fermented vegetables and fermented dairy, such as yogurt and kefir, and miso. Good-quality probiotic supplements are also available, and the best will provide a broad spectrum of bacteria in high quantities. In order for probiotics to flourish, they need to be fed. Prebiotics, which are found mainly in the fiber content of fresh vegetables and fruits, function as food for probiotics. While there is good evidence for the use of a probiotic pill under certain conditions, a diet rich in both probiotics and prebiotics will help you achieve a healthy gut.

form short-chain fatty acids, which provide the necessary fuel for the cells that line the gut wall. The health of the gut wall is crucial for maintaining a healthy immune system. In fact, your gut is the front line of defense when it comes to immune function, so it's in your best interest to nurture the residents living there.

Only in recent years has research into the millions of bacteria within our gut advanced, and with it our burgeoning understanding of how this microbial community governs so many aspects of our health. We are just starting to get a glimpse at how various types of microbes first inhabit and then flourish in our guts, how much variance there is in the types and amounts of microbes among individuals, and how these communities reflect or determine aspects of health that may seem unrelated. Already gut bacteria have been identified as important (alongside other factors) to the risk of cardiovascular disease, arthritis, bowel problems, Crohn's disease, and colitis, and there are recognized links between gut bacteria and obesity, diabetes (types 1 and 2), depression, and non-alcoholic fatty liver disease.[5] People who suffer from these conditions have different bacteria, both in terms of the number of bacteria and the different types, as compared to the bacteria in healthy subjects.[6] Further, it seems that the bacteria actually change before these conditions pop up. In other words, a seemingly fit, healthy, lean athlete is not immune from developing diabetes or another chronic health condition if he or she has a poor diet.

Athletes are less likely to be overweight and sedentary, the most recognized risk factors for diabetes, but research has shown that poor diet is enough to shift an athlete's bacterial population to resemble that of an individual who suffers from the complications of this disease.[7] Antibiotic use has also been shown to effect gut flora, and research is mounting to suggest that use of these drugs is also linked with rising rates of obesity.[8] Antibiotics have long been used in farming to promote weight gain (and profit gain) in animals, so it shouldn't really be surprising that the same is occurring in humans. These facts should make you sit up and take note. What you consume directly affects your health.

Gut bacteria also play an integral role in how we tolerate and react to the foods we eat on a day-to-day basis. Feed them a poor diet, and the troublemakers of the pack will flourish, causing you all sorts of issues. Feed them a nourishing diet and look after them, and they in turn will reward you. Processed carbohydrates and sugars encourage aberrant or less favorable gut bacteria. Different bacteria also digest food differently, with some species gleaning more energy from the same foods than others. In other words, the number of calories absorbed from a meal can fluctuate based on the different gut flora makeup of two individuals. Obese individuals have different microbiota—reduced numbers and diversity—compared to lean individuals, for example.[9]

There are ongoing studies considering the role of gut bacteria in treating conditions and diseases. Some have looked at transplanting different types of bacteria as a treatment for obesity. Fecal transplants, as scary or as odd as they might first seem, have been highly successful in treating certain parasites, and there are current clinical trials showing success for these bacterial transplants in treating severe colitis, which for sufferers has meant years of continual diarrhea, pain, and extensive social anxiety restrictions.[10] Probiotics (sources of beneficial bacteria) and prebiotics (the food supply for bacteria) are also being investigated in supporting good health in a range of ways and with promising results.

In summary, the bacteria in your gut are important and you want to look after them.

UNDERSTANDING FOOD INTOLERANCES

The terms *allergy*, *intolerance*, and *sensitivity* are used interchangeably throughout the medical and nutrition world as well as in more popular articles and health reviews. While there are important distinctions to be made between all three and the physiological responses that accompany them, I think it is important not to get too wrapped up in defining exactly what is meant by *intolerance*, at least in terms of you as an individual and what it means for your diet on a day-to-day basis. The bottom line is this: *You have an intolerance for a specific food if you feel better and notice a decrease in symptoms when you avoid it.* You have a sensitivity to specific foods and ingredients when you are able to tolerate them, but only in limited amounts. In this case, you can decide whether to avoid these foods or eat them in moderation. Whether you are dealing with intolerance or sensitivities, for an athlete, feeling even marginally better can translate to improved training, better recovery, increased mood, and ultimately superior results come race day.

You do not need scientific reasoning, a test, or a diagnosis to make this judgment. If you feel better after eliminating a specific food, you don't need a doctor, nutritionist, or lab technician to confirm your findings. Unless you are dealing with an allergy, which requires vigilance and a thorough understanding of potential sources of contact, it is more important for you to simply avoid certain foods rather than fully understand the scientific reasoning. In some cases, reliable, proven tests or a knowledgeable nutritionist can be very valuable in providing support and helping you navigate the process of identifying problematic foods, pointing out hidden sources and eliminating them while maintaining optimal nutrition. However others simply cannot experience what you are feeling and reporting, so the onus is always on you. There is also no reason to think that any one food is mandatory for you to meet your nutritional goals, so don't be alarmed at having to avoid certain foods or groupings of food. History has demonstrated that humans are very good at surviving and thriving on very different diets. This book will guide you through the process of choosing the foods that are best for you and eliminating those that inhibit performance and optimal health so you can put together your best diet. Just as your training plan will be different from that of your training partner, so too your diet will be unique to you.

IDENTIFYING THE SIGNS OF FOOD INTOLERANCE

Food intolerances may not have the same sense of urgency as allergies do, but the seriousness of a food intolerance shouldn't be underestimated. Over the course of many years or countless exposures, the effects of a food intolerance on your health and body can be uncomfortable, embarrassing, and in some cases, extremely debilitating. We are also seeing increased recognition that inflammation resulting from poorly tolerated foods may contribute to or exacerbate obesity and diseases including heart disease, depression, diabetes, and some cancers.[11]

ALLERGIES *vs.* INTOLERANCE

To understand the seriousness of a food allergy, you only have to think of that kid whose life is threatened by being in the same room as a peanut. In the case of a severe allergy, minuscule exposure is all it takes for the body's immune system to kick into overdrive. Symptoms often occur immediately, and some carry life-threatening consequences: difficulty breathing, skin rashes such as eczema and hives, and vomiting.

Allergies are the result of an overactive immune system and involve activation of either immunoglobulin E (IgE) antibodies or T cells in response to environmental substances or foods that are normally harmless. IgE immune reactions generally occur immediately or within several hours of ingesting the allergen, whereas T cell–mediated reactions can be delayed up to 48 hours. Most allergies present in babies and young children and dissipate by the time the child starts school; however, allergies can present at any time throughout life, even if you have consumed the same foods safely in the past.[12] Among allergy sufferers, there is usually a family history of allergies and presentation of symptoms such as skin eczema, asthma, or hay fever.[13] Professional diagnosis of food allergies is essential in order to avoid confusing severe symptoms with other possible medical conditions. Food allergies require an increased vigilance in comparison to food intolerances because the stakes are higher.

According to the Centers for Disease Control and Prevention, these eight foods account for 90 percent of all food allergies:[14]

Eggs / Fish / Milk / Peanuts / Soy / Shellfish / Tree nuts / Wheat

Gastrointestinal issues are typically considered evidence of a food intolerance. When problems arise, our logical assumption is that "it must be something I ate." However, for the majority of people with food intolerances, gastrointestinal complaints are not present. In these instances, it becomes more difficult to identify the problem or make an association between diet and physical issues that are seemingly unrelated. Food and stomach issues are easily linked, but it's more of a jump for most people to consider that food can impact the brain or the skin or the respiratory system. Instead, they look to other possibilities to explain their symptoms.

Cravings can also be a sign of food intolerance. Sometimes problematic foods give you a "high" because your body becomes somewhat addicted to the hormones histamine and cortisol that are released in response to the aggravating foods. Inevitably, what goes up must come down, and you are likely to experience a very low point after you consume these foods, for example headaches or negative changes in mood. Those feelings, of course, can only be rectified by consuming more of the problem food in order to experience that "high" again. This is the cycle of cravings in motion.

It can be difficult to reconcile that these "feel-good" foods are potentially not good for you. We see this when people go on an elimination diet and initially feel worse. The highs they were getting from problem foods are not there any more. The good news is that if you are truly able to avoid the problematic foods, the associated cravings subside relatively quickly after you remove them from your diet and mood swings and other symptoms are alleviated. One way to pinpoint your own feel-good foods? Be on the lookout for things you consume daily and feel anxious about giving up.[15]

All foods contain chemicals—either natural or artificial or both—and some intolerances are the

TABLE 1. Possible symptoms of food intolerance

BODY SYSTEM	SYMPTOMS
Gastrointestinal	Bloating, diarrhea, loose stools, constipation, stomach cramps, discomfort, gagging, mouth ulcers, bad breath, nausea
Central nervous	Irritability, poor memory, poor concentration, headaches, migraines, mood changes, fatigue, poor sleep
Integumentary (skin, hair, nails)	Itchiness, hives, rash, reddening, flushing, eczema
Skeletal	Muscle pains, joint aches, poor recovery
Respiratory	Wheezing, asthma, hay fever, dripping nose
Urinary	Frequent yeast infection, irritation, frequent need to urinate
Cardiovascular	Feeling faint, palpitations

result of a chemical buildup; in other words, a small amount of the problem food may not produce any adverse effects, but over time and with exposure to either that same food or other foods containing similar chemicals you are sensitive to, a threshold may be reached and symptoms may appear.[16] It's something akin to "the straw that breaks the camel's back." Adding to the chemical load can be sensitivity to nonfood items, such as soap, detergent, or pesticides. This is important to keep in mind. Intolerances caused by chemical buildups can be much trickier to identify. It's not always a simple cause-and-effect relationship.

Food intolerances are highly individual, but many are genetic—they just manifest themselves in different ways. So Grandma's eczema, your dad's irritability, and your own gut pain may in fact be related to the same food intolerance, even though at first glance the symptoms have nothing in common.[17] When I began exploring my own food intolerances, I shared my experiences and knowledge with my family, encouraging them to also try making some changes. My parents are world-champion masters rowers, so they were already eating a very healthy diet and maintaining an extremely high level of fitness. But my dad has suffered from gut issues all his life. Although he realized his problems were probably not normal, he had fully accepted them as his normal. When he eliminated gluten and other grains from his diet, he felt worlds better. Today there is no way you could convince him to eat a piece of bread or tempt him with a cookie. My mum, on the other hand, never had gut issues and was less obviously reacting to any foods in particular. As the cook in their house, it made things easier for her and Dad

to be eating the same foods, so she also embraced a diet free of gluten and grains. She was surprised to find that her lifelong reflux suddenly disappeared. She also dropped considerable weight and went from being a very fit, strong lady to an even stronger, svelte world-champion rower in her sixties, competing at her high school weight.

It is beyond the scope of this book to detail all the factors that can cause, contribute to, or confound suspected food sensitivities, but it's a wide-reaching list that reveals just how intricate our bodies are. When investigating your own food intolerances, you might find that hormones, stress, temperatures, seasons, and other environmental factors play a role.

When considering symptoms and possible intolerances, it's important to keep in mind that food intolerances and allergies can present at any age and can change over time, which is another reason they're sometimes difficult to identify and address. Consider instances where children grow out of certain allergies or a food intolerance or allergy is introduced by a parasite or after a severe illness. Food intolerances can also occur during or after pregnancy, likely due to hormonal changes in the body.

WHY FOOD INTOLERANCES GET MISSED

Most food intolerances go undiagnosed for many years.[18] It's quite common for the symptoms to go unnoticed because people either learn to get by or assume that their discomfort is "normal," especially if tests and doctor visits have failed to discover any other reasons for their symptoms. Food intolerances may also be difficult to identify or diagnose because they can take some time to present. While allergic reactions are immediate, some symptoms of food intolerances may not be noticeable until up to 72 hours later. In this time you are likely to have eaten a wide range of foods and so finding the actual culprit food is a challenge. Complicating things further, symptoms often overlap with other conditions, and problematic foods cause different symptoms in different people. In my own case, I was able to make a connection between gluten consumption and persistent headaches and "brain fog," but for another person an intolerance could appear as gastrointestinal problems such as bloating or diarrhea.[19] This is why many intolerances typically go unrecognized, especially if the advising doctor or specialist does not identify the link between the gut and other bodily systems.

I often meet with clients who have come to conclude that they are intolerant of a certain food or food group based on a simple cause-effect investigation. Sometimes they are right, but given the delay involved with food intolerance, the process is usually more complex. For instance, if you are plagued by stomach issues following your morning latte or bowl of cereal, it is not unreasonable to assume that you are intolerant of dairy. You might eliminate dairy and notice that the majority of your symptoms disappear. But if you still don't feel 100 percent, it may in fact be gluten that you are intolerant of. Gluten sensitivity leads to inflammation throughout the gastrointestinal tract, where the lactase enzyme that digests the milk protein lactose is found. This means that you might still be unable to properly digest or tolerate dairy, but dairy is not the primary cause of the problem. With a proper elimination diet you could identify foods containing gluten as the primary culprit. You might even find that by avoiding gluten, with time you are able to once again tolerate dairy because the lactase enzyme is restored.

Fear can also delay the identification of a food intolerance or stand in the way of implementing a diet free of suspect foods. Many of us cannot or do not want to accept that our symptoms could be caused by something that we eat. It would be easier if there were a medical explanation, a prescription, or even a procedure that would make us feel better. The thought of not being able to eat a favorite food can cause anxiety, especially when family traditions and customs are concerned. What will your Italian grandmother think when you tell her that you can no longer eat her homemade ricotta ravioli because you are lactose intolerant? The support of family and friends will help you invest in the process and stick to any changes you need to make, even if this means sitting your family down and explaining to them what you are doing and how they could best help you. After all, it would be

FEAR can also delay the identification of a food intolerance. …
Many of us cannot or do not want to accept that our symptoms could be caused
by something that we eat.

easier to resist tiramisu if your nonna wasn't pushing it down the table.

WHY FOOD INTOLERANCES ARE ON THE RISE

Evidence shows that prevalence of both food allergies and intolerances is growing worldwide. Because diagnosis is difficult and many people simply self-diagnose, it is really hard to get a handle on the true numbers of food allergies and intolerances to gauge just how common they are globally and how quickly they are increasing.[20]

In particular there has been a clear increase in celiac disease numbers that goes well beyond improved diagnosis. Back in the 1950s, over 9,000 U.S. Air Force recruits had samples of blood taken to test and screen for streptococcus. Little did anyone know at the time that these men and their blood samples would become famous within the world of celiac disease research. More than 50 years later, researchers uncovered these well-preserved blood specimens and decided to test for the prevalence of celiac disease in comparison to present-day numbers. The results showed a 4.5-fold increase in rates of the disease, suggesting that whatever has happened to cause these rapid changes has been environmental.[21]

Specialists confirm that they are seeing more people with celiac disease, but gluten sensitivity is also becoming more prevalent. Thanks to consumer demand for fluffy bread and the ingenuity of selective breeding, the gluten content of modern wheat and other grains has increased substantially. While this might seem like a minor issue, when you

consider how frequently most people eat wheat products, even a small increase in gluten content means that overall consumption is amplified over the course of a day, a week, a year. Recent studies have shown that symptoms of patients suffering from irritable bowel syndrome (including frequent constipation and/or diarrhea, cramping, bloating, pain) improved when their diet shifted from modern wheat-based foods to foods that use an ancient form of the grain.[22] Inflammatory markers also decreased along with symptoms, highlighting the fact that modern-day versions of commonly eaten foods are different from the older varieties. We have also shifted from more traditional methods of preparation—for example, the slow and unhurried process through which sourdough bread has traditionally been made—to faster, more cost-effective methods that use yeast and other artificial rising agents. Unlike modern methods, the natural process of fermentation reduces the gluten content of the final product. Consequently, we are being exposed to gluten in higher quantities than ever before, and this exposure may be to blame for the rise in the numbers of people being diagnosed or identified as gluten intolerant. Looking beyond gluten, all the evidence points to the fact that both allergies as well as intolerances are on the rise. The question is why.

One important piece of the puzzle is our changing food environment. Our food sources have evolved rapidly and significantly to be vastly different from those of our grandparents, not to mention their grandparents. Looking back to past generations, these time frames are but a blink in terms of *Homo sapiens'* evolutionary history, but if we were to compare diet over the last 50 years

How EXTERNAL FACTORS
exacerbate or cause INTOLERANCE

Stress. The strong connection between the gut and mind plays an important role in the presentation and severity of symptoms. Consider stress management and other lifestyle factors along with dietary changes.

Alcohol. Irritants such as alcohol can increase permeability of the gut wall, changing how we are able to deal with foods.

Weakened immunity. Because the gut is the command center for the body's immune defenses, any time the immune system is challenged by infection or illness, the gut's ability to cope with digestion and maintenance of the gut barrier may be compromised.

Hygiene. Exposure to unsanitary conditions or poor hygiene will introduce lots of foreign and unwelcome critters that place stress on the immune system, again affecting how smoothly the gut functions. On the flip side, our obsession with cleanliness as a society means that our immune system can be kicked into overdrive when it encounters something that should actually be considered harmless.

Vitamin D. Research shows that vitamin D may influence how the immune system functions and the health of the cells in the gut as well as the body. This is why we see a direct correlation between low levels of vitamin D and many conditions and diseases.

Gut bacteria. The types and size of bacterial colonies in your gut can change as a result of your diet and use of antibiotics. As gut bacteria evolves, it will affect how food is digested and how healthy the mucosal barrier is, potentially leading to new symptoms or changing the severity of existing symptoms.

Parasites. Physical damage and changes to gut bacteria can also be caused by parasites, which can be very hard to identify and get rid of. This is a concern that should be addressed with a medical professional.

WHEN INVESTIGATING your own food intolerances, you might find that hormones, stress, temperatures, seasons, and other environmental factors—even chemicals such as cleaning products and perfumes—play a role.

there would be some stark differences. Engineered breeding and corporate farming have become the norm, influencing what ends up on our plate. Our diet is confined to a more limited number of foods—and hugely reliant on wheat, corn, fructose, and soy, all of which can cause inflammation and may contribute to development of intolerances.

In addition to allergies, food sensitivities also seem to be increasing, with more and more people being diagnosed or figuring out for themselves that certain foods just don't sit well with them.[23] Whether this is a true rise in the prevalence of food sensitivities or merely a rise in awareness is difficult to ascertain.

ATHLETES & FOOD INTOLERANCE

It's very common to see athletes eating gluten-free, avoiding dairy, and eliminating grains or other foods—and not because they have celiac disease or an allergy, but because they perceive that their performance improves with these restrictions. Sometimes this is a short-term measure focused on particular competitive goals, for example making race or competition goal weight, but in other cases these choices are lifestyle changes rooted in improved well-being.

Although there is no evidence to suggest that the prevalence of food intolerances in the athletic population is any different from that of the general population, athletes may be more likely to either identify or be diagnosed with a food intolerance. For an elite athlete, improvements in mere seconds, milliseconds, and percentages add up to a significant difference in overall performance, so identifying the cause of anything that reduces the capacity to compete, train, or recover is worth pursuing. Diet is paramount for everything from the ability to recover from hard training to hand-eye coordination and quick reflexes to building a body best suited to the demands of a particular sport.

Athletes are more likely to recognize symptoms of food intolerance, largely because they are used to analyzing how they are physically performing and feeling, so they may also be more attuned to things going awry or being slightly off. Symptoms of food intolerance may also be more pronounced or frequent with the effects of exercise, prompting athletes to seek out a diagnosis or probable cause.

Furthermore, increasing permeability of the gut will also increase the risk of food intolerance. As the gut becomes more permeable, the body's immune system is activated to deal with the invading foreign particles. There are three main ways in which the gut can be compromised during exercise: the physical and mental stress associated with intense training or race day nerves, the mechanical factors related to the motion or activity of exercise, and the dietary intake and medications that are often the mainstays of athletic populations.

Because these factors lead to the onset of food intolerance symptoms, we need to differentiate between the possible causes: a food intolerance that is *exacerbated* by exercise; a food intolerance that is *caused* by exercise; and symptoms such as GI distress that may present themselves like food intolerance when they are actually *related to the effects* of exercise itself. For instance, too much fiber or a state of dehydration can cause GI distress during a workout. It has nothing to do with a food intolerance. Understanding how exercise impacts your gut will help you begin to determine whether you need to avoid certain foods altogether, limit your intake of a particular food prior to training, or simply change your fueling strategy.

STRESS

Everyone experiences stress, whether physical, mental, or emotional. An athlete experiences every form of stress in competition or during intense training, and many of the body's systems are affected, including the cardiovascular, endocrine, muscular, urinary, and gastrointestinal systems. The athlete's gut is particularly susceptible to stress, whether that stress stems from a workout or life in general.

Acute situational stress that makes it hard to stomach food—you've likely experienced this kind of stress on race day or during a job interview—is one thing. Ongoing or chronic stress, such as you might experience under consistently high training loads or when dealing with financial or personal difficulties, also affects gut function. Family or job stress, fatigue, lack of sleep, reduced immunity, illness, and injury are all forms of stress that impact how your body functions.

These stressors can disrupt the intestinal lining and trigger inflammation leading to either an exacerbation of symptoms or the increased likelihood of experiencing symptoms.[24] It's crucial to understand this when considering the impact of exercise on food intolerance in athletes. For instance, we know that stress associated with competition—wanting to perform well, striving to reach goals, or being fearful of not meeting the expectations of a coach or teammate—can increase sensitivity when it comes to intolerance to particular food chemicals.

Physical stress associated with hard-working athletes also has consequences when it comes to immune system function and in turn the ability to deal with particular foods. Reduced immunity is quite common in athletes. When you are training hard and constantly pushing your physical boundaries, you can find yourself forever on the brink of illness. Research shows that although exercise in general boosts the immune system's defense capabilities, overtraining diminishes these returns. Even in healthy athletes, the immune system is temporarily depressed in the hours following an intense workout.[25] Since the majority of the body's immune system originates in the gut, it follows that a compromised immune system also entails compromised gut function and/or the integrity of the gut's mucosal barrier—that "brick wall" separating the external from the internal. A compromised gut barrier means that food particles may be able to enter the bloodstream more readily, triggering the body's immune defense and causing undesirable symptoms—in other words, food intolerances. It could be the case that you are dealing with an underlying food intolerance that is made worse with training or an intolerance that is only present with the added stress of training.

pregnancy.[46] The likely explanation is that these intolerances, especially if undiagnosed or poorly managed, contribute to nutrient malabsorption, particularly of iron, zinc, and folic acid, which are essential for reproduction, the immune system, and energy production.

Women who are not aiming to get pregnant, whether in the near future or ever, still want to ensure that their bodies are functioning well. The same holds true for men. Alterations in hormonal function are not desirable from either a sports performance perspective or a bigger picture of health.

COMMIT TO FINDING YOUR BEST FOODS

Figuring out exactly what your best foods are is an ongoing process that begins with cleaning up your diet and addressing any existing food intolerances. Simply managing your symptoms will eventually lead to more widespread problems and negative consequences for your body. What seems minor today can become much more serious if left unchecked. Why take that chance? It could also be the case that you have a food intolerance without obvious symptoms. You will need to be your own advocate and do some experimenting to find out exactly what your body needs to feel great and compete at your full potential. This book will guide you through the process and give you the nutritional background you need to find your best foods. What you eat and how you treat your body will pay dividends in all aspects of your life, both now and far into the future.

FIXING
YOUR DIET

When it comes to food, there is no one diet that works well for everyone. The best diet for you does not necessarily match any strict, universal rules. No experimental data or research can account for every single person; what works is highly individual and may require some experimentation on your part.

There are three initial steps for finding your best diet. These steps will help guide through the process of identifying the foods that promote better health and performance for you.

The first step is to **eliminate unhealthy foods**. There are some foods that humans have a low tolerance for—in other words, in larger quantities, or when consumed frequently, these foods cause health to deteriorate and accelerate disease. Foods that detrimentally change how the human body functions could be termed "common" or "shared" food intolerances. These foods do not support optimal health or, as a consequence, optimal performance for the athlete. If the foods we eat compromise maximal efforts and acute performance along with recovery and immunity, either directly or indirectly, then it is impossible to achieve peak personal excellence or reach a new personal best in sport.

More and more, chronic inflammation is being recognized as the root of many common health problems rather than merely a symptom. Inflammation has been found to precipitate or accelerate a broad range of health conditions and diseases, from obesity, depression, certain cancers, heart disease, gastrointestinal issues, reduced life span, and diminished quality of life.[47]

However, inflammation is not all bad. It's a natural defense mechanism to address acute injuries and attacks on the body. Immune cells and key nutrients are sent to the sites of injury or infection, and the healing process begins. But when inflammation becomes chronic, pervasive, or out of control, damage is done. Chronic inflammation can be blamed on lifestyle: stress, lack of sleep, environmental pollutants, smoking, lack of exercise, and of course diet. There are also certain foods that are known to increase inflammation, and others that help curb it.[48]

Sugar, refined or processed carbohydrates, and refined fats and oils are the worst dietary offenders when it comes to inflammation.[49] And yet it's surprising how many athletes rely on these types of foods to help fuel their training. Some athletes believe that exercise counters the negative effects of these foods, so they feel they have earned the right to indulge. In other cases, athletes are simply eating the foods labeled as "sports nutrition." Whether as a result of misinformation or clever marketing, we buy into the notion that such foods and drinks are necessary. I am in no way suggesting that all sports foods have no place in the athlete's diet, but they must be chosen and used selectively and be well-timed. Avoiding the foods that have been proven to cause inflammation will promote well-being and support optimal training and racing.

The next step in choosing your best diet is to **eliminate or minimize the specific foods that could possibly be causing intolerance symptoms.** This second category of food intolerances is highly individual. There are more nuances to how dairy, fructose, gluten, food chemicals, and other specific food proteins and carbohydrates react in the body. Each individual will have different symptoms and thresholds of tolerance. Take two people with a gluten sensitivity or intolerance: For one person, the sensitivity may present as stomach pain and bloating and occur with even a trace amount of gluten, for example in a sauce or some confectionary that is not obviously made from gluten. The second person may suffer from a mild rash that crops up three days after eating a bagel for breakfast and a dinner of pizza washed down with wheat-based beers. Both people may have genuine reactions indicating gluten intolerance, and yet the second person seems to have a higher threshold for the amount he or she is able to consume before paying the price. The base functional diet allows you to carefully observe how your body responds to different foods by first simplifying what you are eating. By using a food diary to record any symptoms that occur, you can identify the foods you are intolerant of.

The final step in this process, after you have identified your intolerances and allowed your gut to heal, is to **reintroduce as many healthy foods as possible that are well tolerated.** Again, your food diary will be critical in ruling out particular intolerances and sensitivities. The goal is to have the greatest possible variety in your diet. Not only is variety healthy in terms of nutrition, it's also optimal in terms of feeling satisfied and enjoying food in the long term.

AVOID THE UNHEALTHY FOODS THAT CAUSE INFLAMMATION

The average American eats close to a ton of food every year.[50] That is a lot of food and a lot of opportunities to choose foods that support a happy, healthy, functioning body. Unfortunately, our burgeoning waistlines and increasing health care costs make it clear that most Americans are not faring so well.[51] When unhealthy foods make up a significant portion of your diet, they bring negative implications for health and athletic performance by increasing chronic inflammation. These are the foods that should be eliminated from, or at least minimized in your diet:

> Processed and packaged foods
> Refined grains
> Sugars and sweeteners
> Trans fats, hydrogenated oils, and some animal fats
> Artificial colors and flavors

This might look like a short list, but the reality is that most foods consumed in the Western world comprise one or more of these types of food. The prevalence of these foods in our diet is problematic. If you were to eat a food that falls into one of these categories on occasion or in very small quantities, it's likely that it would have no detrimental effect. Issues arise when you habitually eat these foods.

USDA data illustrates that we are spending the vast majority of our food budget on unhealthy foods. Americans spend over 30 percent of their consumed-at-home food expenditure on either refined grains or sugars. Another 10 percent is spent on beverages (many of which are sweetened and not included in the sugar category, since they make up such a large proportion just by themselves), and a further 10 percent goes toward frozen or premade meals. At the same time, there is a high amount of fresh food waste in the home; of the approximately 10 percent spent on fresh fruits and vegetables, much ultimately goes uneaten—instead left to spoil in the back of the crisper before being tossed into the trash.[52] How does your household food budget compare?

PROCESSED & PACKAGED FOODS

If asked to think about all the foods available to eat in the world, you might think that there is an endless variety. And indeed we are surrounded by choices that are expanding every day. In fact, in the U.S. market alone more than 20,000 new food products are introduced onto supermarket shelves every year. More than 25 percent of these are either confectionary or snack products, and a further 20 percent fall under the beverage category.[53] While we find ourselves staring at a seemingly endless variety of foods in the grocery store, the diversity of the foods we eat is actually surprisingly small. You might think that one food is different from another, and yet on closer examination you will likely find that the ingredient lists are extremely similar.

Corn, soy, wheat, or a derivative of one of these ingredients are present in so many processed and packaged foods that even if we opened a different package for each meal, the majority of our calories would come from the same limited sources. It's hard to believe, but almost 40 percent of an average American's daily recommended intake of calories comes from soy and corn alone, and most of this is consumed in the form of either added sugar (high-fructose corn syrup) or added fat (soybean oil). One or the other or both are added to virtually all processed and packaged foods.[54]

Over 77 percent of all processed foods have sugar added to them, and that does not include naturally occurring sugars, only *added* sugars. The average American consumes a staggering 150 pounds of sugar per year, while the average male teenager downs 34 teaspoons per day, mostly in the form of soda and other sweetened drinks, including sports drinks.[55] Next time you're in the supermarket, read the product labels. Even foods you don't consider sweet are likely to have added sugar, including breads, sauces, crackers, cereals, pickles, and mayonnaise.

REFINED GRAINS

Wheat is another diet staple, with the average American consuming over 130 pounds of this grain annually in the form of cakes, cereals, breads, cookies, and crackers, all of which are highly refined products.[56] Why are grains such as wheat so prevalent? Because they are cheap and relatively stable, which allows them to be effectively stored. Unlike fresh produce, grains are less prone to volatility in pricing and availability due to fluctuations in weather. Plus, they can be used in combination with other inexpensive products (think vegetable oils like corn and soy) to make an endless variety of food. Throw in a little coloring here and a little flavoring there, along with plenty of preservatives, and those refined-flour products can take on any number of guises in the supermarket aisle. And so while we may feel as though we are eating different foods, the ingredients label and statistics on consumption tell a different story. This lack of variety and exposure to different foods is thought to be one possible explanation for the rise of food intolerances. Insofar as the food industry offers less diversity and quality, it is partially to blame for the fact that intolerances are becoming more common.

Grains such as bread and pasta are carbohydrates that the body quickly converts to sugar to be used for energy in the body. Excess consumption is associated with higher levels of inflammatory markers.[57] This is especially problematic for athletes because the common wisdom is to eat lots of carbohydrates, and nutrition plans are often packed with these types of foods: cereals for breakfast, sandwiches for lunch and snacks, pasta for dinner with a side serving of bread to further boost carb intake. Aside from the potential for inflammation, high refined carb intake prevents us from eating more micronutrient-rich and anti-inflammatory foods—after all, there is not that much room left for salads and vegetables after all those grains are consumed. Even when a high-carbohydrate intake is required, there are better options than refined-grain products.

An emphasis on a diet high in carbs may be warranted at certain times, particularly for athletes consistently training hard, but it often filters down to those who participate in sport or who exercise, even if very infrequently or at low levels of intensity. Everyone likes to view themselves as an athlete no matter their level of training or accomplishment, and that attitude can be used to justify unhealthy nutritional choices despite having very different requirements.

SUGARS & SWEETENERS

Athletes may be healthier than the population in general, but highly processed and refined carbs and sugars still form a significant part of many athletic diets, whether in the form of specialized sports foods (drinks, bars, chews, and gels) or as justifiable reward: ice cream with a cookie for dessert, a post-run brownie, or that mid-afternoon iced caramel latte before an evening workout. Let's be honest, it's easy to make these choices knowing that the extra calories will soon be burned off in a workout. That philosophy might hold up if you are only concerned with your outward appearance and body weight, but excess sugar is problematic for more than its potential to make people fat; it's also linked with increased mortality rates.[58] So regardless of body weight and body fat, what you eat does matter.

Hormone receptors located in the gut respond to what we eat. Certain foods, especially sugar, may trigger responses that act on the brain in an addictive fashion. The catchphrase of the nutrition world has long been "everything in moderation," but for some people it's impossible to eat just a little of something. Just a taste can spiral into over-eating, especially in the case of sugary and refined

Spotting SUGAR

It's not as easy as it sounds! Manufacturers often use alternative forms. Here are some of the most common types to look for:

The "-ose" suffix. Sucrose, maltose, dextrose, fructose, glucose, galactose, lactose, high-fructose corn syrup, glucose solids

Syrups and sweeteners. Cane juice, dehydrated cane juice, cane juice solids, cane juice crystals, dextrin, maltodextrin, dextran, barley malt, beet sugar, corn syrup, corn syrup solids, caramel, buttered syrup, carob syrup, brown sugar, date sugar, malt syrup, diatase, diatastic malt, fruit juice, fruit juice concentrate, dehydrated fruit juice, fruit juice crystals, golden syrup, turbinado, sorghum syrup, refiner's syrup, ethyl maltol, maple syrup, yellow sugar

The "-itol" suffix. Generally denotes a sugar alcohol. Maltitol, sorbitol, xylitol. These sweeteners might be calorie-free, but there is evidence to show that they are just as bad (if not worse) than real sugar. Furthermore, sugar alcohols are often poorly absorbed, leading to symptoms of intolerance.

foods. In an evolutionary sense, these energy-dense foods were once in short supply, and as a survival mechanism people were inclined to stock up when they became available. In our modern world we are surrounded by easily obtained foods, and these "survival" cravings are actually to our detriment. The consequences are easy to see in our modern landscape. While our response to sugary and refined foods might not fit the standard definition of food intolerance, we'd all be better off if we reduced or eliminated them from our diets.

Excess sugar causes inflammation, damages blood vessels, alters gut microbiota, and results in myriad other negative health effects.[59] Artificial (nonnutritive) sweeteners, which have been shown to alter insulin and blood glucose levels, disrupt the lining of the gastrointestinal tract and negatively affect the composition and numbers of gut microbiota.[60] There are times when sugar is unavoidable and even beneficial for athletes (explained more in Eating for Performance, page 85), but on a day-to-day basis sugar intake needs to be minimal. An athletic body battling inflammation from a suboptimal diet is never going to provide the best platform for solid training and racing performance.

TRANS FATS, HYDROGENATED OILS & UNHEALTHY FATS

Omega-6 fats are essential within the body, but most people get far too many of them in their diet, tipping the ideal ratio of omega-6 and omega-3 fats too far in favor of the more inflammatory omega-6s. Found in vegetable oils such as corn and soybean oils as well as seed oils (cottonseed, etc.),

omega-6 fats are used in almost all processed and packaged foods, as well as being the popular choice for many restaurants. By contrast omega-3 fats, known to dampen inflammation, are primarily found in fatty fish such as salmon and sardines and in nuts such as walnuts, and are more desirable and elusive in average diets.[61]

Animal fats, although natural, can also be problematic if the animals are not fed a healthy diet. If humans experience inflammation from foods that we are not designed to eat in large quantities, it makes sense that the same would hold true for animals. Let's follow that logic. Cows naturally eat grass, not corn and other grains. When cows are fed a grain-based diet, they get fat. Fat cows benefit both the farmers, who are paid by the pound, and the consumers who demand lots of cheap meat, but the cows are not necessarily healthy. Because toxins are stored in fat, when we eat animal fat from a not-so-healthy animal, we increase our own risk of inflammation. Not only is there more fat in a grain-fed animal, the fat composition of animals actually changes based on the farming methods that are used to raise them. A grass-fed cow will provide meat that is naturally high in anti-inflammatory omega-3 fats, but if the cow is switched to a grain-fed diet, omega-6 fats soar.[62] Interestingly enough, grass-fed beef has as much omega-3 fat as salmon, a fish famed for its omega-3 content.

ARTIFICIAL COLORS & FLAVORS

Anytime you see artificial colors and flavors in a list of ingredients it should be a huge red flag. These additives are designed to mimic flavors

TABLE 2. Inflammatory foods: The worst offenders

FOODS	WHAT'S ON THE LABEL	WHY TO AVOID IT
TRANS FATS		
Processed foods, fast foods and snacks, margarine, shortening	Hydrogenated or partially hydrogenated fats	Triggers inflammation, raises LDL cholesterol
SUGAR		
Processed food and snacks, beverages, fruit juices, sports drinks, cereals, granola bars	Fructose, sucrose, glucose, maltose, (look for "ose" at the end) plus corn syrup, rice syrup, fruit juice concentrate, maltodextrin, malt syrup, sugar alcohols (xylitol, sorbitol, mannitol), agave syrup, maple syrup, honey, high-fructose corn syrup	Promotes inflammation, damages blood vessels, alters gut microbiota, promotes myriad other negative health effects throughout the body
ARTIFICIAL SWEETENERS		
Processed food and snacks, beverages	Aspartame (NutraSweet, Equal), saccharin (Sweet'N Low), acesulfame potassium, sucralose (Splenda), neotame, nonnutritive sweeteners	Alters insulin and blood glucose levels, disrupts the lining of the gastrointestinal tract, and negatively affects the composition and number of gut microbiota
ARTIFICIAL FLAVORS & COLORS		
Seasoning mixes, processed foods and snacks, beverages, canned soups and soup mixes, deli meats, salad dressings	Numbers! Some of these are natural, but most are artificial. Also look for MSG, sulfates, benzoates, flavor enhancers, stabilizers.	Excitotoxins in artificial colors and flavors induce inflammation.
REFINED GRAINS		
Breads, bagels, pasta, crackers, tortillas, cereal, etc.	Enriched flours, flour(s), starches (e.g., wheat, corn), corn flour	Refined grains quickly convert to sugar, and excess consumption of refined grains is associated with higher levels of inflammatory markers, linked with escalating rates of obesity and other chronic inflammatory conditions.
PROCESSED MEATS		
Sausages, deli meats, bacon	Nitrates, sulfites, preservatives, MSG	Contain additives, which are among the most common sources of chemical intolerances. Diets high in processed meats are linked to increased risk of cancer, especially colorectal cancer, and heart disease.
FATS FROM GRAIN-FED OR INTENSELY FARMED ANIMALS		
Beef, chicken, pork, lamb, eggs, dairy products	Grain-fed diet, cage eggs. If grass-fed or free-range isn't specified, it's likely a grain-fed, intensely farmed animal.	They are higher in omega-6 fats and a higher concentration of residual toxins is stored in the fats.
EXCESS OMEGA-6 FATTY ACIDS		
Corn, soy, cottonseed, safflower, sunflower, grapeseed, peanut, and vegetable oils	Nitrates, sulfites, preservatives, MSG	Omega-6 fats are essential, but modern diets provide too much omega-6 and not enough omega-3 oils, triggering inflammation.

TABLE 3. Inflammatory foods: The other offenders

If you have individual allergies, intolerances, or sensitivities, the following foods will also cause inflammation, either by irritating the gut or by triggering an immune response.

FOODS	WHAT'S ON THE LABEL
DAIRY—CASEIN OR LACTOSE	
Milk, cheese, ice cream, yogurt, sour cream, cream, butter, ghee, recovery and protein drinks/shakes. Processed food and snacks also often include dairy, as do baked goods.	Lactose, lactate solids, lactalbumin, lactoglobulin, whey, casein and caseinates, milk, milk solids
GLUTEN	
Breads, pasta, flour tortillas, soy sauce, barley, rye, spelt, durum, faro, semolina, sauces and gravies, thickeners, coating mixes, batters and fried foods, seasoned meats, salad dressings, soups, potato chips/fries, croutons, beer, and potentially in oats and processed foods via cross-contamination.	Gluten, wheat, wheat derivatives, seitan, wheat starch, modified wheat starch, malt, malt extract, malt flavor, malt syrup, brewers yeast
SOY	
Tofu, tempeh, natto, soy milk, soy cheese, soy yogurt, soy bacon/turkey products, meat substitutes, miso, edamame, recovery/protein drinks, plus most processed and packaged foods, including sauces, dairy foods, baked goods, breaded foods, thickeners, drinks	Soy, soybean oil, lecithin, soy sauce, textured soy protein, hydrolyzed vegetable protein, vegetable oil
CORN	
Corn, corn chips, popcorn, corn tortillas, grits, polenta, tamales, cereals, many processed and packaged foods	Vegetable oil, corn oil, corn flour, cornmeal, corn sugar, corn extract, maize flour, corn starch, glucose syrup, corn syrup, fructose syrup, dextrose, dextrin, maltodextrin, xantham gum
YEAST	
Breads and cereals, beer, wine, and ciders, stock cubes, salad dressings, sauces, fermented foods, dried fruit	Yeast, yeast extract
INDIVIDUAL ALLERGENS	
The most common are shellfish, eggs, milk, peanuts, soy, sesame, tree nuts	By law, these are required to be listed on packaging. Also be aware of cross-contamination when dining out.
FOOD CHEMICALS—SALICYLATES, GLUTAMATES, AMINES	
Additives and preservatives, as well as a wide range of natural and fresh foods	Depends on individual intolerance. See page 61 for a more detailed list.
ALCOHOL	
Wines, beers, spirits	Alcohol

and colors found in nature, and also to hide less appealing ones resulting from the process of refining, extruding, and adding ingredients—which removes any of the goodness from the original food. These chemicals make things look better, taste better, and last longer. But put simply, these additives are not food, and what they are added to in most cases could barely be called food either. In fact, in some instances the result cannot legally be called what it is masquerading to be, for example the mayonnaise that can't be called mayonnaise and is instead called "dressing" or the cheese that must be called "processed cheese food." Because of all the extra additives, the final product is far removed from an actual natural food. Aside from these issues, artificial colors and flavors (and even natural added ones) are known to cause allergic and nonallergic reactions. These intolerances are explored more in Target Common Intolerances and Sensitivities, page 48.

While none of the foods mentioned above are ideal, one-off exposures or consumption in very small quantities is unlikely to cause problems for the majority of us. Where issues arise, either in the short term or over a lifetime, is when our diets rely heavily on these foods. Unfortunately, as we have seen the typical diet is made up of these inflammatory foods from the breakfast table right through to dinner, including our snacks and even the sports foods we consume as we strive to get fitter, faster, and healthier. By simply avoiding the foods that cause inflammation, you are likely to feel better.

GET YOUR FILL OF **HEALTHY FOODS**

It's quite possible that the unhealthy foods I've described make up a fairly big chunk of your diet. It's time to fill the gap. The following are the food categories that should form the basis of your diet: fresh produce; nuts and seeds; fresh meats, fish, poultry, and eggs; and natural fats.

FRESH PRODUCE

We have all been told to eat our vegetables from a very young age. Perhaps you love your vegetables and are one of the smart few who regularly fit in the recommended five servings a day. But the majority of people fall short of that target. Well, it's time to fall in love with your greens (and oranges, yellows, reds, blues, and purples), or at least learn how to enjoy them so that they become an abundant part of your meals every day. They will truly love you back.

Think of the produce on display at your local grocer or farmers market. All of those different colors represent different antioxidants and flavonoids. *Antioxidants* is likely a word you have heard before and associate positively with health, specifically with the reduction of inflammation.

In normal day-to-day living, we produce oxidants, or free radicals (unstable molecules), every time we breathe or move. The process of oxidation in the body is like metal rusting. Unstable molecules are very reactive and can result in weakened cell membranes, acceleration of the aging process, and increased vulnerability to diseases. While some oxidation is normal and even necessary for healthy functioning, antioxidants, which are supplied by your diet, help to neutralize excess free radicals and prevent them from causing damage to cells and tissues. A generally healthy body can handle normal levels of free radicals; however, depending on your lifestyle and what you expose your body to, you can overwhelm the ability of antioxidants to counter free radicals' effects. Excessive production of free radicals has been linked to damage and disease including heart disease and cancer. Our modern environment might be particularly harmful—

pollution, pesticides, and smoke are all known to increase the production of free radicals. This makes the importance of a diet rich in antioxidants even more compelling.

So where are antioxidants found? Vitamins A, C, and E along with the minerals copper, selenium, and zinc are common sources. However flavonoids and phytochemicals (plant chemicals that act as antioxidants) present in fruit and vegetables are believed to have even stronger antioxidant effects.

Flavonoids are generally what give plants their different colors, and although about 4,000 types of flavonoids have been identified, researchers admit that we are nowhere near to uncovering all the different types of flavonoids found in plant foods,

TABLE 4. Foods that reduce inflammation

	BEST CHOICES
Vegetables	Dark, leafy greens (kale, spinach, collard greens), cruciferous vegetables (broccoli, cauliflower, cabbage), colorful vegetables (beets, bell peppers, tomatoes, sweet potatoes), garlic, onions
Fruit	Berries (blueberries, strawberries, cranberries, raspberries), tart cherries
Herbs	Basil, parsley, rosemary, oregano
Protein	Fatty fish (salmon, mackerel, sardines, tuna), oysters, organic-pastured meats and eggs
Nuts & seeds	Walnuts, almonds, flax seeds, chia seeds
Spices	Ginger, turmeric, cinnamon
Natural fats & oils	Olive oil, walnut oil, flaxseed oil, macadamia nut oil, avocados and avocado oil
Tea	Green tea, white tea, black tea, herbal teas
Probiotics & prebiotics	Fermented foods (kimchee, kombucha, kefir, yogurt) and supplemental probiotics, fiber

as well as understanding their associated benefits. Regardless, the evidence is pretty clear that a diet high in plant matter is a healthy one.[63] And yet there is also evidence that the benefits from plant antioxidants do not extend to antioxidant supplements. The bottom line is that we would all benefit from eating lots more fruits and vegetables, in a variety of colors.

NUTS & SEEDS

Nuts and seeds are another rich source of antioxidants, and they also have other healthy benefits. Packed with fiber, healthy fats, protein, vitamins, and minerals, nuts and seeds have been linked to longevity. Nuts make an easy, transportable snack, which is good news because studies have shown that people who consume a daily handful of nuts live longer and healthier lives.[64] Nuts, nut flours, and nut butters can also be incorporated into baked goods, main dishes, smoothies, dips, and condiments. Their combination of fiber, protein, and fat might help us moderate our appetite, a notion that is backed up by research.[65]

FRESH MEAT, FISH, POULTRY & EGGS

We tend to think of these foods as being protein foods. And yet they contain so much more that can contribute to ongoing health and optimal functioning. Iron, zinc, iodine, phosphorous, copper, potassium, essential fatty acids, and vitamins are all found in meat and eggs, and are just one of the

CHOOSING YOUR NUTS

If you are looking for the best bang for your buck when it comes to nuts, here are some front-runners:

Walnuts. These brain-shaped nuts are a smart choice because they have the highest level of antioxidants as well as omega-3 fats.

Almonds. Almonds contain the most fiber, helping keep you feeling full and feeding those healthy bacteria in your gut. They are also a good source of the antioxidant vitamin E, and contain some calcium.

Brazil nuts. These nuts are the best dietary source of selenium, a mineral that might help prevent certain cancers.

Macadamia nuts. Macadamia nuts provide a good source of healthy fats as well as fiber, magnesium, calcium, and potassium.

reasons to include these animal foods in your diet. B vitamins, including B12, are only found in animal foods, and the iron and zinc these foods contain are more readily used by the body than iron and zinc from other sources.

Just as a variety of fruits and vegetables helps meet nutritional needs, a variety of meats, fish, poultry, and eggs is beneficial, as each has different nutritional profiles:

> Red meats, including beef, lamb, deer, and bison, offer the best sources of iron, as well as B vitamins (in particular B12).

> Poultry and pork are also good sources of B vitamins, as well as phosphorous and iron, though in lower amounts than red meat.

> Fish and seafood have their own claim to health fame. Omega-3 fats and other essential fatty acids are common in many fish, especially cold-water fish. Vitamins D and A, along with iodine, potassium, and zinc, are also nutrition stars.

> Organ meats, including liver, are actually the richest sources of many nutrients, especially B vitamins and iron, but also vitamins A and D. Organ meats used to be prized for their rich nutritional benefits (and, indeed, in many non-Western cultures they still are), but we seem to have become increasingly squeamish about our cuts of meat. If you want to really boost your nutrient levels, then be brave and seek out some quality liver or other organ meat and give it a try (do get a good recipe, though, as these meats are definitely stronger in flavor, often smell, and can be more difficult to work with. But they're definitely worth it.)

Guidelines for a HEALTHY DIET

Eating well is all about replacing unhealthy foods with the foods that are best for your body.

○ Eat fresh, organic produce. By making an effort to eat what is in season, you will naturally eat a wider variety of foods over the course of the year and also boost nutrient quality.

○ Look for organic grass-fed meat, free-range poultry, and wild-caught or sustainably farmed seafood.

○ Eat plenty of healthy fats.

○ Buy local when you have the opportunity.

○ Avoid processed and packaged foods, refined carbohydrates, and processed oils.

To eat better as a vegan or vegetarian, the same principles for a healthy, anti-inflammatory diet apply, along with a few more:

○ Prepare both grains and legumes (as tolerated) properly by soaking and thoroughly cooking them.

○ Use supplements as needed, especially if you are vegan. Stay on top of potential deficiencies with periodic blood work.

Remember that nutrition is personal. Each and every person responds differently to food and has different needs. Figure out if your body reacts negatively to any foods and eliminate them, or eat them only in tolerable amounts.

> Eggs can truly be classified as a superfood. They contain all the essential amino acids along with vitamins A, B12, D, E, niacin, the minerals copper, iron, sulfur, and phosphorous, as well as essential fatty acids.

Diet and lifestyle are clearly important for humans, and they are also important for animals: An animal that has led a happy, healthy life produces healthy meat (and/or eggs).

NATURAL FATS

The first myth to dispel is the notion that fats make us fat. Despite their unfair name and vilification in the past, fats play a vital role in our health. We need fats for our brains and nervous systems, energy production and transport, hormone production, cell membrane integrity, and digestion. Simply put, we cannot survive without fat. But it is important to eat the right fats. Trans fats and excessive amounts of omega-6 fats are unhealthy options that you should avoid. So what about saturated fats, which have long been labeled as the "bad" fat? Although the accepted wisdom had been that saturated fat causes heart disease, the latest and largest meta-analysis of published evidence throws this advice into doubt.[66] Indeed, no benefit was found to support cutting back on saturated fats, nor was there any support for replacing saturated fat with the unsaturated mono- or polyunsaturated fats.[67] The word *saturated* refers simply to the structure of the fat, which is very stable and not prone to oxidation. Unfortunately, the misleading information that inspired so many people to reduce saturated fat typically resulted in them replacing it with carbohydrates, often in the form of highly processed sweet foods that amplify inflammation and other health risks.

Essential omega-3 fats, on the other hand, have been widely recognized as beneficial to health. They act as anti-inflammatories that counter the much more prolific and pro-inflammatory (and yet still essential) omega-6 fats. There are plenty of other types of fats, but rather than thinking of fats as being either good or bad based on whether they are saturated or unsaturated, mono- or poly-, simply concentrate on incorporating more high-quality natural foods that contain fats into your diet.

VEGAN & VEGETARIAN DIETS

There is little doubt that vegetables play a vital role in health. Among popular diets widely credited with conferring health benefits—Mediterranean, Paleo, Japanese—plant foods are the common theme.[68] In fact, a good vegetarian diet has many things going for it: It is likely higher in fiber, and being rich in fruits and vegetables means it is rich in vitamins, especially vitamins C and E. Vegetarians also avoid some of the worst offenders of the modern food world: processed meats (i.e., deli meats) as well as meat from animals that have been intensively farmed. But simply avoiding animal meat doesn't constitute a healthy diet. Because there are a lot of valuable nutrients available in food that comes from animals, being vegetarian requires a conscientious approach to keeping your diet well balanced for health and performance. And the potential for food intolerances remains, however navigating them is more complicated when meat is excluded from your diet.

Some people will choose to follow a vegan or vegetarian diet for personal, ethical, environmental, cultural, religious, and other social reasons. I respect these decisions, and it is not my business to dissuade anyone from those beliefs. But if you restrict your diet to vegetarian or vegan foods based on the belief that it is *healthier*, rest assured that you can safely return to the butcher or fishmonger. Studies showing that red meat brings negative health consequences and increases the risk of cancer stem from research that has lumped quality steaks with processed hot dogs doused in condiments! Making a conscientious effort to eat healthy grass-fed or wild-caught meats has in fact been proven to be beneficial to health.

While vegan diets have long enjoyed the halo of being healthy, there are some key nutrients that are almost impossible to get in a diet that eschews all animal proteins. Perhaps this is because as omnivores we need some of our nutrients to come from plant foods, others from animal foods. Should you choose to avoid animal foods, pay particular attention to the following key nutrients: calcium, iron, zinc, vitamin A, vitamin B12, vitamin D, omega-3 fatty acids, and protein (depending on the requirements and composition of your diet).

Because these nutrients are mostly found in animal foods, supplementation might be required to meet adequate levels with a vegetarian or vegan diet. Vegetarians who eat eggs and dairy (as tolerated) will find it easier than vegans to meet some key nutritional targets.

TARGET COMMON INTOLERANCES & SENSITIVITIES

Now that you've eliminated all the unhealthy foods that we're all intolerant of and replaced those nutrition sources with healthy foods, it's time to eliminate (at least temporarily) other foods that could be causing problems for you. This is the second step toward establishing a base functional diet. Once you've eliminated these possible sources of inflammation and have been eating a base functional diet long enough to give your system time to heal and reset, you will reintroduce these foods one at a time to see what effect they have on you. In Identifying Your Intolerances (page 69), I'll give more details on specific diet questions and the reintroduction process.

GLUTEN

Walk down virtually any aisle of any supermarket and you will find a growing number of gluten-free products. Of course, the food industry both drives the movement and responds to consumer demand,

but this rise in commercially available products is nevertheless telling. The quality of these products is questionable and their necessity even more so—have you ever studied the list of ingredients on some foods labeled gluten-free? They might be found in the health food aisles, but that doesn't give them a free ticket to be considered healthy foods.

Indeed the explosion of products and numbers of those eating gluten free has caused others to question the legitimacy of the gluten-free movement. To what extent are people jumping on the bandwagon as they do with other diet trends, either to lose weight or, as some cynics have postulated, merely to gain attention? We do know with certainty that both celiac and non-celiac gluten intolerance are real and serious conditions. Furthermore, the number of people who suffer from these conditions is greater than what we might think and continually growing.[69] It's important to figure out if you are someone who would benefit from avoiding gluten.

The protein gluten, comprised of peptides glutenin and gliadin, is found in wheat, rye, barley, but also in ancient grains such as spelt and kamut. Gluten is what gives the springy elasticity to bread and provides cakes and other baked goods with their texture and consistency.

When someone who is intolerant of gluten eats a piece of bread (or any other food containing gluten), the gut identifies the gliadin component as a threat. Antibodies are produced and sent out to fight off this attack. Unfortunately, to the antibodies, gliadin looks similar to some body tissues, and so these tissues also get attacked. Imagine a village of red hat–wearing people happily going about their business. The chief spots an invader wear-

ing a blue hat and commands his soldier to go and deal with the blue-hatted threat. The soldier happens to be color blind, so instead of just attacking the blue-hatted invader, he also attacks his own villagers who are wearing hats, albeit red hats. He cannot tell the difference. This attack makes the villagers angry, and they turn on each other, arguing and fighting among themselves. They are no

SOURCES OF GLUTEN

Wheat and wheat derivatives including: Wheat berries, durum, emmer, semolina, spelt, farina, faro, graham, kamut, einkorn wheat

Rye, barley, triticale, brewer's yeast

Malt, including: Malted barley flour, malted milk or milkshakes, malt extract, malt syrup, malt flavoring, malt vinegar

Other common gluten-containing foods: Pasta and noodles, breads, tortillas, and wraps, cereals, crackers, cookies, and other baked goods, beers and other fermented beverages, potato chips and fries (gluten is in the batter or malt ingredients), sausages and other processed meats (gluten is in the starch used), soy sauce (use tamari instead), candy, energy bars and granola bars, sports bars, some processed foods (from cross-contamination)

List adapted from The Celiac Disease Foundation, www.celiac.org

longer able to do their jobs properly, and the village is no longer productive. To make matters worse, they are now vulnerable to other invasions—the green and yellow hats seize their opportunity and step right on in.

For people with celiac disease and gluten sensitivity, a similar scenario is played out in their gut—although to greater and lesser degrees depending on where they fall on the spectrum. Gliadin is identified in the gut by the immune system as a poten-

Guidelines for a HEALTHIER GUT

A healthy gut means eliminating the foods that are causing inflammation but also being kind to your gut to allow it to recover and repair. Time is part of the equation, but these other dietary and lifestyle habits are also key.

○ Stick to anti-inflammatory foods for the majority of your dietary intake. Inflammatory foods kill off good gut bacteria and encourage growth of bad bacteria.

○ Incorporate more fermented foods (e.g., kombucha, sauerkraut) and probiotics into your diet. Research shows that probiotics help maintain healthy gut bacteria populations and the overall integrity of gut barrier function, thus preventing leaks and reducing the risk of toxins entering the bloodstream and thereby inflammatory reactions and food intolerances.[70]

○ Prebiotics, a fancy word for the fibers found in plant matter, are just as important to provide food for the probiotics. Stock your diet with vegetables, fruits, and nuts to provide lots of fermentable fiber, which will serve as food for the probiotics.

○ Only use antibiotics as needed, and avoid animal products that have been exposed to antibiotics.

○ As an athlete you can encourage a healthy population of bacteria within your own gut by steadily building fitness and not overreaching. Appropriate workouts

and timing will help facilitate positive acute stress that induces adaptation, allowing you to become fitter, faster, and stronger and strengthen your immune system. But the chronic stress that can occur with overtraining, inadequate recovery, or trying to achieve too much before you are ready for it can compromise body functions and structures, including that of the digestive tract and the resident bacteria.

○ Stay hydrated. Adequate hydration helps maintain the gut wall's cellular structure (important as a barrier) as well as its function.

tial threat. Antibodies are produced in response and attack these invading proteins; however, they also attack transglutaminase, the enzyme secreted by the intestinal wall to aid with digestion. Transglutaminase also helps hold the gut wall together, so when it is attacked the mucosal barrier becomes compromised. This results in that leaky gut, where foreign particles entering the body trigger an immune response that results in systemic inflammation.[71] It is important to distinguish between celiac disease and other forms of gluten intolerance, as one requires strict adherence to a gluten-free diet for life, and the other is likely to be a little more forgiving in terms of vigilance and tolerance levels and may also be dependent on other external factors.

CELIAC DISEASE

Celiac disease is an non-allergic autoimmune reaction to the protein gluten—found in wheat, barley, and rye—which causes inflammation and damage to the microscopic villi that line the intestine. Villi are vital for nutrient absorption. These fingerlike projections increase the surface area of the intestine, effectively capturing more nutrients in the process. When a person with celiac disease eats foods with even trace amounts of gluten, the villi are flattened and left unable to properly absorb nutrients. Think of a nice thick shag rug that suddenly becomes worn and threadbare. Left untreated, celiac disease can lead to devastating nutritional deficiencies including anemia (reduced iron absorption) and osteoporosis (reduced calcium absorption). Consequently, bone loss and/or injury in the form of repetitive stress fractures or osteopenia, as well as symptoms of low iron such

as fatigue, poor immunity, and healing, are commonly seen in those diagnosed with celiac disease. Sufferers may also complain of stomach pains or diarrhea, but perhaps more often there are no gastrointestinal complaints at all. This is one reason many people with celiac disease go undiagnosed.

Blood tests are used to screen for celiac disease, but the results are often inconclusive or give false results (false positives as well as false negatives). To date, the definitive diagnosis comes from a bowel biopsy that involves an endoscopy to examine the extent of damage to the villi. For those who experience reactions to gluten, the process of diagnosis can be frustrating and painful as well as cause further damage, as the testing requires the consumption of significant amounts of gluten-containing foods for a period of time. For people who have already eliminated wheat and are feeling better, participating in testing can be a hard decision to make, so they often self-diagnose gluten intolerance.

NON-CELIAC GLUTEN INTOLERANCE OR SOMETHING ELSE?

The term *gluten sensitivity* is often used to explain or define a situation where someone does not have celiac disease or an allergy to gluten, and yet he or she feels distinctly better when avoiding wheat and other gluten grains. They may not have the intestinal damage that elicits a celiac diagnosis, but report improved energy, recovery, and healing when gluten is removed. These non-celiac gluten sensitivities are now broadly recognized among medical and scientific communities.

However, when it comes to gluten intolerance—and intolerances or sensitivities in general—

we are only just beginning to scratch the surface in our understanding of these interactions between food and body. What is commonly called gluten sensitivity may not be due to gluten at all.

Grains, both those with gluten and those without, contain any number of other proteins and compounds. Gluten just happens to be the one that is most recognized now. But while we may be good at identifying gluten in a scientific sense, our bodies are not always that good at picking it out from other proteins. This means that for those sensitive to gluten, including some with celiac disease, it is not enough to simply avoid gluten; other grain proteins may be good enough impersonators of gluten that our bodies cannot see through the disguise and mount a reaction of the same force and destruction against these proteins as they do against gluten. For those individuals, the end result is the same: damage and inflammation, and confusion as to why they do not seem to improve even when eating strictly gluten free.[72]

Perhaps in the future reliable tests will enable us to pinpoint exactly which proteins we are intolerant of and which grains are necessary for us as individuals to avoid. For now we may not be able to identify these particular proteins, but the treatment remains the same: removal of the foods that make us feel worse.

In addition to people with gluten and other grain protein reactions, there are some who will feel better when they avoid eating bread and pasta for different reasons. Despite the belief that they are gluten intolerant, their issue might in fact stem from the types of carbohydrates found in these foods. In some people, certain carbohydrates can be malabsorbed in the intestine, leading to fermentation in the bowel and inducing symptoms easily confused with gluten intolerance.[73] These carbohydrates, known as FODMAPs, are discussed more later in this section.

DAIRY

Dairy is another food that is ubiquitous in the Western diet. In fact, most countries recommend that people eat at least two servings per day; however, dairy foods remain a common source of both allergens and intolerances. The main problems stem from either reactions to lactose, the carbohydrate found in dairy, or casein, one of the dairy proteins.

LACTOSE INTOLERANCE

Lactose is a sugar carbohydrate found exclusively in animal milk products such as milk, yogurt, cheese, and ice cream. Lactose digestion requires the enzyme lactase in order to break down lactose into smaller simple sugars for absorption. All human babies have lactase enzyme in order to digest their mother's milk, but the enzyme usually decreases by around age 5. The lack of this enzyme and therefore the inability to properly digest lactose-containing foods triggers symptoms including diarrhea, stomach pain, and bloating.

However, certain populations have maintained the lactase enzyme, thus allowing them to consume dairy foods as an important food source. Essentially, maintaining the enzyme is a genetic mutation that became advantageous for survival.[74] Northern Europeans as well as descendants from

certain parts of Africa, the Middle East, and central Asia continue to express the enzyme lactase into adulthood. Other populations, though, including African Americans and those of Asian descent are almost all lactose intolerant.[75] Indeed, lactose intolerance is probably one of the most prevalent food intolerances worldwide, so dairy is most definitely one of the first foods to consider when looking at potential sources of food intolerances.

In those individuals who are missing the lactase enzyme, lactose enters the gut but is too large to be absorbed, so it can give rise to symptoms. Lactose intolerance may also be influenced by volume or the amount eaten, with small amounts posing no problems for people but large or frequent consumption bringing on the symptoms.[76]

Even for those who are generally able to digest lactose, intolerance can be transient or pop up under certain circumstances. Since lactase is produced by the epithelial cells lining the gut wall, damage to the gut can disrupt production of this enzyme. Damage can occur because of irritants, antibiotic use, stress, celiac disease, changes in gut flora, food poisoning, or viruses.[77] With the removal of the particular irritant, dairy foods may be able to be reintroduced and be well tolerated by someone who previously though they were off limits as the primary cause of their symptoms.

Milk and ice cream contain the highest amount of lactose. Other dairy products such as yogurt, kefir, and cheese are made through the process of fermentation, which decreases their lactose content. Butter is perhaps the lowest lactose-containing dairy product, so many people who are unable to tolerate milk find they can tolerate butter in their diet.

CASEIN & WHEY

Often people assume that their reaction to dairy is because of lactose, but they could instead be reacting to one or more types of casein. Casein is the protein found in cow's milk and is known to be one of the most common allergens. Whey is another dairy protein, and although it can also be the source of an intolerance, this is much more rare.[78]

Symptoms of casein intolerance and lactose intolerance can be similar, and given that most dairy foods contain both components in varying amounts, it can be difficult to pinpoint if it is the protein (casein) or the carbohydrate (lactose) that is the problem. In reality, it might not matter—you can test specific foods (i.e., yogurt vs. milk vs. cheese vs. butter) for yourself and see how you react. For some, all dairy is fine. For others, only hard cheeses and fermented yogurts can be tolerated in small amounts due to their lower lactose content. Still others will find that all cheese gives rise to symptoms because of the casein or perhaps the naturally occurring chemicals. Some individuals find that even butter or whey protein powders cause them upset. By testing your diet carefully, you should be able to discover what foods you can consume and how much. Even if you need to avoid dairy completely, you can still get all the nutrients you need.

WHAT ABOUT CALCIUM?

Dairy is a rich source of calcium, which is important for tooth and bone strength and health, as well as muscle contraction and other bodily functions. Dairy also provides a good source of nutrients, including protein and vitamin D. But there are plenty of populations that have not traditionally eaten dairy and yet have low rates of osteoporosis,

clearly demonstrating that dairy is not essential to bone health and achieving adequate levels of calcium. Asian populations are an obvious example. They have high levels of lactose intolerance, minimal dairy consumption (in traditional diets), and low rates of osteoporosis compared to Western populations that, despite high dairy consumption, have the highest rates of osteoporosis.[79]

Prevention of osteoporosis depends on building strong, dense bone during your first 30 years of life. After this time, bone density gradually declines, so it's important to limit the bone loss experienced in adulthood. Building and maintaining bone density relies on good nutrition that includes calcium, vitamin K, and adequate vitamin D, as well as weight-bearing activity. Vitamin K is found in leafy greens such as kale, Swiss chard, broccoli, spinach, and parsley, and vitamin D is found in fish liver oils, fatty fish (salmon, mackerel, tuna, sardines), egg yolks, cheese, and liver, with the best source of vitamin D being sunlight.[80]

TABLE 5. Top non-dairy sources of calcium

FOOD / SERVING SIZE	CALCIUM (mg)
Collards *1 cup (190 g) cooked*	357
Rhubarb *1 cup (240 g) cooked*	348
Sardines *3 oz. (85 g) canned*	325
Spinach *1 cup (180 g) cooked*	291
Turnip Greens *1 cup (144 g) cooked*	249

Source: USDA database

FODMAPS

When we eat foods containing carbohydrates, a portion is not absorbed or digested in the small intestine and instead passes right on through to the large intestine, where it ferments and produces short-chain fatty acids and gas. This is a normal process that occurs in everyone. In fact, the short-chain fatty acids are an important part of a healthy digestive system because they provide fuel for gut bacteria and help protect the mucosal lining of the intestines. However, in some people certain carbohydrates eaten in threshold amounts can lead to symptoms such as bloating, gas, distension, abdominal discomfort, and either diarrhea or constipation, or a mix of both.

The bacteria residing in your gut will determine how you handle and respond to these particular carbohydrates. For some of us, any amount is absolutely fine, while others can consume only a minimal amount before they encounter symptoms, the severity of which may range from mildly annoying to debilitating. For those facing less severe symptoms, it's common to accept them—when you are accustomed to the discomfort it's easy to assume that everyone else is dealing with similar feelings.

The types of carbohydrates that are most commonly malabsorbed in the intestine are known as FODMAPs (fermentable oligosaccharides, disaccharides, monosaccharides, and polyols). These are simply the technical names for the structure of the sugar molecules (*saccharides* is another name for sugar). All carbohydrates are broken down into glucose or sugar molecules through digestion.

TABLE 6. Common high-FODMAP foods & sweeteners

FODMAP	FOODS
Excess fructose	**Fruit:** Apples, mangos, pears, watermelon
	Sweeteners: Corn syrup solids, high-fructose corn syrup, honey
Fructants	**Vegetables:** Artichokes, asparagus, beets, chicory, dandelion leaves, garlic, green onion (white part), leek, lettuce, onion, onion powder, raddicchio
	Grains: Rye, wheat
	Food chemicals: Inulin fructo-oligosaccharides
Lactose	**Dairy products:** Condensed milk, custard, dairy desserts, evaporated milk, ice cream, margarine, milk, milk powder, soft unripened cheeses (e.g., ricotta, cottage, cream, mascarpone), yogurt
Galacto-oligsaccharides	**Legumes:** Baked beans, bortolotti beans, garbanzo beans (chickpeas), kidney beans, lentils
Polyols	**Fruit:** Apples, apricots, avocados, cherries, longon, lychee, nectarines, pears, plums, prunes
	Vegetables: Mushrooms
	Food chemicals: Isomalt (953), maltitol (965), mannitol (421), sorbitol (420), xylitol (967)

Source: Monash University. "Monash University Low FODMAP Diet Booklet," 3rd ed. Melbourne: Monash Univ., Dept. of Gastroenterology, 2015.

FODMAPs are found in a wide variety of foods: fruits, vegetables, grains, legumes, dairy, nuts, and seeds. Apples, pears, onions, garlic, wheat, and rye are among the common culprits. Given that FODMAPs describe only certain carbohydrates, proteins and fats are free of them.

HOW DO I KNOW IF FODMAPS ARE A PROBLEM FOR ME?

Avoiding FODMAPs is gaining recognition as a successful way to bring relief to people who suffer from irritable bowel syndrome (IBS), ongoing GI symptoms that remain unexplained or without an identifiable cause. It is important to understand that while avoiding FODMAPs can help control IBS symptoms, *FODMAPs are not the cause of an irritable bowel.*[81]

The standard FODMAP diet, developed by Australian research scientists at Monash University, eliminates *all* foods containing these specific carbohydrates for a period of six to eight weeks and then tests you for each individual group to determine which carbohydrates you might be sensitive to.[82] This process can be tricky, as you must remember

TABLE 7. Finding alternatives to high-FODMAP foods

FOOD	HIGH-FODMAP FOODS	LOW-FODMAP FOODS
Vegetables	Asparagus, artichokes, beets, celery, garlic, leeks, legumes/pulses, onion and garlic salts, onions (all varieties), savoy cabbage, sugar snap peas, sweet corn	Alfalfa, bean sprouts, bok choy, bell peppers, carrots, chives, choy sum, cucumbers, fresh herbs, green beans, lettuce, tomatoes, zucchini
Fruits	Apples, mangos, nashi pears, nectarines, peaches, pears, plums, watermelon	Bananas, grapes, mandarin oranges, melons, oranges
Nuts & seeds	Cashews, pistachios	Almonds (handful), pumpkin seeds

Source: Monash University. "Monash University Low FODMAP Diet Booklet," 3rd ed. Melbourne: Monash Univ., Dept. of Gastroenterology, 2015.

exactly which foods contain FODMAPs. It can also lead some people to turn to gluten-free foods, which may be highly refined and/or high in sugar. Either way, it's a solution that can lead to still more inflammation and add nothing in the way of nutrients.

I recommend that you take an easier approach, at least initially: Eliminate grains, legumes, and dairy foods. Because these foods are generally high in FODMAPs, for the majority of people total consumption of any FODMAPs is brought down below a threshold level, meaning that symptoms are likely to be relieved. This allows you to continue to eat the more nutrient-dense fruits and vegetables, even those containing FODMAPs, and is an easier diet to follow, rather than trying to remember which fruits and vegetables should be on or off the table.

If you find that even after avoiding grains, legumes, and dairy you continue to have GI symptoms such as bloating, diarrhea, constipation, distention, abdominal pain, and discomfort, it is possible you have a high level of sensitivity to FODMAP foods. You may need to experiment with reducing the higher FODMAP–containing fruits and vegetables and instead focus on the alternatives outlined in Table 7.

FRUCTOSE

Fructose is one of the FODMAP carbohydrates, but it deserves special mention based on the prevalence of fructose in sports foods. It is also important to distinguish between fructose intolerance and fructose malabsorption. The former is a rare and life-threatening condition where the liver lacks a specific enzyme and hence the body is unable to process fructose or convert glucose into glycogen. Fructose intolerance demands strict avoidance of fructose, and failure to avoid it can lead to coma, seizures, and even death. If you are looking to explain your mild gastrointestinal issues, rest

assured that it is unlikely that you have fructose intolerance. However, fructose malabsorption is much more common.

Under normal circumstances, fructose is absorbed through the gut wall and transported to the liver for processing. However, sometimes a particular protein needed for this transportation is missing, and fructose sugars end up in the large intestine instead. Here they ferment via the action of the resident gut bacteria, producing gas with bloating, diarrhea, flatulence, and the urgency to rush to a bathroom. Some degree of fructose malabsorption may be present in as much as 30–40 percent of the population. When you consider that sports foods and drinks often use fructose as a carbohydrate source, they could potentially be of concern for many athletes and to blame for some instances of GI distress.[83]

The inability to process and absorb fructose can be hereditary but can also be exacerbated or brought on by other circumstances:

> The total amount of fructose consumed at any one time.
> Whether glucose is consumed in conjunction with fructose. Glucose assists in transporting fructose sugars across the gut wall, leaving less to ferment in the intestines.
> Whether celiac disease, which increases the potential for fructose malabsorption, is present.
> The type and number of gut bacteria, which will affect the way fructose that ends up in the large intestine is processed.
> Whether other food intolerances that damage or irritate the gut wall make it more likely fructose will be malabsorbed.

SOY

Soy is another food that is high on the allergen list and is also strongly linked to food intolerance. Thanks to subsidized production, soy is an inexpensive filler, and it also works well as a carrier for other flavors. Soybean oil is omnipresent. In fact, if you ate out today, you most likely ate foods cooked in soybean oil. If your food came out of a package, you probably consumed soy. Approximately 60 percent of all packaged foods contain soy in some form—soybean oil, soybean protein, soy lecithin, textured vegetable protein, or hydrolyzed vegetable protein.[84] Our overconsumption of soy in these forms has the potential to increase inflammation and may also contribute to rising rates of allergies and intolerances as previously noted.

Proponents of soy often point to the famed health of the Japanese people and their typical diet. And it is true that the Japanese have been among the longest living, with some of the lowest rates of cardiovascular disease, obesity, and diabetes.[85] (It's worth noting that these rates are increasing rapidly due to the influx of Westernized foods and the fast-food culture that is changing the food landscape.) It is also true that for centuries the Japanese diet has contained soy. However, Americans commonly consume soy very differently from the Japanese, a fact that should bring us to question the promotion in the United States of foods like soy milk as healthier alternatives. Traditional Japanese forms of soy—tofu, tempeh, natto, and even traditional soy sauce—are all fermented. Fermenting changes the structure of the proteins and begins to break down the carbohydrates. Additionally, in

Japan soy is used more as a condiment than as the meal itself, so the total amount of soy consumed as part of a Japanese diet is quite modest.[86] This is in contrast to the unfermented soy that Westerners consume in much larger quantities. Unfermented soy is high in FODMAPs and, as mentioned earlier, is a common ingredient in processed and packaged foods—and may be a major contributor to symptoms in some FODMAP-sensitive individuals.

There are other contentious issues linked to soy consumption. Production of soy is notoriously mired in genetically modified organisms (GMOs). Furthermore, soy contains phytoestrogen, chemicals that mimic female sex hormones and have been linked to reproductive and hormonal issues in both men and women. However undesirable you find these issues, neither one strictly factors into intolerance, but they're worth noting. In summary, there are compelling reasons to limit or avoid soy, regardless of whether you feel FODMAPs are an issue for you.

FOOD CHEMICALS

This next category of food intolerances is more pertinent to those who are symptomatic, especially if symptoms are not confined just to the gut but involve other areas of the body and/or mind. Even if you haven't personally experienced a negative reaction to food chemicals, it's worth being aware of the potential risk involved.

We tend to think of chemicals as cleaning products or perhaps as additives such as artificial flavors and colors. But all foods contain chemicals, even fruits and vegetables, proteins and fats, and other foods usually considered healthy. Some chemicals are clearly beneficial, such as vitamins, and others are toxic to humans: fertilizers, strong cleaning agents, and chemical weaponry, for example.

Salicylates, amines, and glutamates are common chemicals found in a wide range of substances, including foods, either in artificial, added forms (additives) or as naturally occurring chemicals. In fruits and vegetables, these chemicals act as natural pesticides, deterring would-be predators as well as disease and bacteria. As such, they are usually concentrated in the epidermis, or "skin," and just below the outer leaves, bark, roots, and seeds. Other common nonfood sources of these chemicals are cleaning and cosmetic products as well as aspirin (salicylates). For athletes, many sports foods and drinks contain chemicals, both naturally and as additives. When you think about the time you are most likely to consume these foods in large quantities—in and around competition day—you can see that an adverse reaction would not be ideal for performance.

Although all people will react to some degree to these food chemicals if their exposure or consumption is high enough, some are more sensitive than others. How sensitive you are depends on how much of the chemical-containing foods you can tolerate. Once your threshold amount is reached, the buildup of chemicals irritates nerve endings throughout the body, giving rise to myriad unpleasant symptoms. Usually foods contain more than one type of chemical in varying amounts, and the amount can even change according to how ripe or "aged" a food is. For instance, before a tomato is ripe it is high in salicylates. As it ages, amines and glutamate levels rise and salicylates fall.

FIGURE 1. Cumulative effect of some food intolerances

Each spike represents a food eaten. Some meals do not result in any symptoms but add to the total load in the body. Other foods or meals tip over the threshold level and result in symptoms.

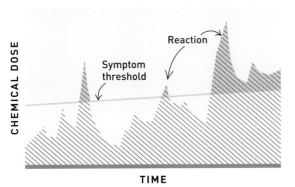

SALICYLATES

In large enough doses, salicylates are toxic for everyone. Everyone has his or her own threshold, but if you are extremely sensitive, you need to strictly avoid particular foods and food groups that contain salicylates. For some people a reaction may not occur immediately after ingestion, but with repeated exposure the chemical builds up. It is only with this cumulative effect that a threshold is reached. For these people, managing tolerance and symptoms is not a matter of eliminating any particular foods, but rather being mindful of the *total* consumption of *all* of the foods that contain the offending chemical.[87]

The range of symptoms is broad and includes physical as well as mental and behavioral issues. Interestingly, much of the research on these intolerances stems from linking children's behavior to certain foods and food additives. Because children are much smaller than adults, they are more sensitive to smaller doses of these chemicals, so thresholds are reached more readily.[88] Symptoms linked with salicylate sensitivity include the following:[89]

> Itchy skin, hives, or rashes; eczema; acne; mouth ulcers; sore, itchy, puffy, watering, or burning eyes
> Stomach pain or upset stomach, diarrhea, nausea, bloating, constipation
> Asthma, breathing difficulties, persistent cough
> Headaches and migraines, dizziness
> Fatigue, lethargy, insomnia, sleep disturbances
> Aching muscles and joints
> Constant hunger, excessive thirst, food cravings
> Sensitivity to light and noise
> Unexplained weight gain/loss
> Depression, anxiety, poor self-image
> Hyperactivity, lack of focus
> Irritability, mood swings, anger, and/or behavioral problems
> Brain fog, confusion, poor concentration
> Panic attacks and phobias

AMINE/HISTAMINE

Histamine is produced by the body as part of an allergic reaction. It is also naturally present in some types of foods, in which case it is more commonly known as an amine. This is why a histamine intolerance or sensitivity is also known as an amine sensitivity.

Amines form naturally in foods as a result of the fermentation process breaking down particular proteins. Fermented, aged, cured, and pickled foods are generally high in amines, including cheeses, cured or aged meats (fresh meats and fish are free from amines), alcohol, soy sauces, yeast, chocolate, sauerkraut, and tinned meats and fish. Some fruits and vegetables are also relatively high in amines, including ripe tomatoes, eggplant, and spinach.[90] See the sidebar on page 61 for a list of foods high in amines.

Generally, humans produce an enzyme called diamine oxidase that breaks down the amines in foods as they enter the digestive system. When people are deficient in this enzyme, the amines remain at levels that induce symptoms such as wheezing, runny nose and eyes, rashes, itching, diarrhea, vomiting, and pain. Women are more at risk for sensitivity to amines because of their inter-action with estrogen. Fluctuations in levels of estrogen throughout the monthly cycle may also mean that symptoms are heightened at certain times.[91]

As with other enzyme deficiencies, those with poor gut health or other food intolerances that have damaged their membrane barrier or those who have aberrant microbiota are more at risk of suffering from amine sensitivity. This is because the enzyme necessary to break down amines is found in the membranes of cells lining the wall of the small intestine and upper large intestine. By removing gut irritants and inflammatory foods from your diet and allowing the gut to heal and healthy bacteria to flourish, tolerance to amines may return or at least improve.[92]

If you discover or suspect that you are sensitive to amines, consult with your doctor because there are certain medications that interfere and interact with the production of diamine oxidase.

GLUTAMATE

Glutamates are found naturally in most foods and form the building blocks of proteins. They are also known as the flavor enhancers of the food world. Monosodium glutamate (MSG) is both a human-made as well as a natural additive used in many foods to enhance flavor. Foods naturally rich in glutamates include cheese, mushrooms, yeast, soy

THE FAILSAFE DIET (Free of Additives, Low in Salicylates, Amines, and Flavor Enhancers [glutamates]) was developed by Australian researchers specifically for these types of chemical food intolerances. If you are continuing to struggle with symptoms even after trying the base functional diet, then the FAILSAFE diet and associated resources are a great reference point. A strict elimination diet that looks at these food chemicals will also involve looking at medications and exposure to other chemical sources such as cleaning products, perfumes, and lotions. One-on-one help with a nutritionist or dietitian might also be useful to ensure that you are eating adequately. Be aware that some of the foods allowed within this diet are low in nutritional density (e.g., refined grain products and packaged foods), and I would recommend avoiding them as well.[93]

Common sources of FOODS NATURALLY HIGH IN CHEMICALS

If you have a sensitivity to food chemicals, the base functional diet will help you determine which foods are okay to eat and in what amounts. The list below provides examples of the foods highest in naturally reactive chemicals.[94] Many foods have not yet been tested for chemicals, which means you can only know if a food is problematic through trial and error.

Salicylates. All herbs and spices, including cardamom, coriander, cumin, ginger, paprika, turmeric, and peppermint; coffee, herbal tea, and tea; apricots, cantaloupe, cherries, citrus fruit, dried fruit, fruit juices, nectarines, peaches, strawberries, watermelon; tomatoes and tomato sauces; asparagus, avocado, bell peppers, chili peppers, Chinese spinach, choy sum, cucumber, eggplant, fava beans, olives, onions, and zucchini; stocks, pickled vegetables, and vegetable juices

Amines (generally strong-tasting foods). Alcohol, cocoa, and dark chocolate; fully ripe bananas; almonds, broccoli, mushrooms, and pickles; aged or cured meats and cheeses; fermented foods and sauces such as sauerkraut, soy sauce, and yeast; fresh pork; canned fish; oily fish (salmon, sardines, tuna)

Additional chemicals to look for (may be present even in foods such as dairy, dried fruits, or supplements).
Colors: All artificial colors, annatto coloring 160b

Synthetic antioxidants: 310–312, 319–321
Preservatives: 200–203, 210–218, 220–228, 249–252, 280–283
Flavor enhancers: 600 numbers

Natural monosodium glutamate (MSG). Present naturally in cheeses, meat extracts, mushrooms, soy sauce, tomato paste, and yeast

Note: For an updated list of the most recently tested foods, visit the Australasian Society of Clinical Immunology and Allergy (ASCIA) web site, www.allergy.org.au.

Foods low in natural food chemicals:

Bamboo shoots / Brussels sprouts / Butter (preservative-free) / Cabbage / Celery / Chayote / Cheese / Chives / Cream / Eggs / Fresh fish (except salmon, shrimp, and tuna) / Fresh meats / Garlic / Green beans / Iceberg lettuce / Leeks / Milk / Mung bean sprouts / Parsley / Pears (Packham and Bartlett) / Potatoes / Red cabbage / Rutabagas / Shallots

sauce, tomatoes, and various sauces—all strongly flavored foods. As with salicylates and amines, sensitivity depends on cumulative ingestion or exposure to glutamates rather than an isolated episode.

While it is possible to have a reaction to any one specific food chemical, sensitive individuals will often react to the accumulation of *all three* food chemicals: salicylates, amines, and glutamates.[95] The base functional diet I present in this book is a great starting point for anyone with symptoms who is trying to pinpoint culprit foods. Because food chemicals are more highly concentrated in processed foods, even those sensitive to these nat-ural food chemicals may find that by eliminating processed and packaged foods their tolerance threshold is never breached and so symptoms are relieved.

For those very sensitive individuals who continue to have symptoms after eliminating these foods, it may be necessary to look at limiting consumption of some natural, healthy foods as well. These individuals (and particularly children) might need further assistance in implementing a low-chemical diet. It is a complex undertaking, and support is warranted, especially if you find you need to eliminate lots of fruits and vegetables.

OTHER TYPES OF INTOLERANCE

ALCOHOL INTOLERANCE

This is actually a genetic condition whereby individuals are unable to break down alcohol in the liver. Symptoms such as facial flushing, feeling hot, headache, or stomachache, as well as increased heart rate and nasal congestion can ensue. This intolerance should be more readily diagnosed, seeing as most people don't drink as often as they eat foods. But because wine, beer, and other alcoholic drinks can also be sources of gluten, wheat, and amines and other food chemicals (in the form of preservatives), they can irritate the membrane of the gut, leading to more widespread inflammation, with some individuals being more sensitive than others. This is why you won't be drinking alcohol on a base functional diet.

Be aware that even if you do not have a specific intolerance, heavy or frequent drinking can lead to inflammation and scarring of the liver (known as alcoholic hepatitis and cirrhosis respectively) and high blood pressure. Even in moderate amounts, alcohol also can increase the risk of certain cancers.

GUT IRRITANTS

Caffeine and spices such as chili and curry can act as irritants that give a "hurry up" signal to the contents in your gut, manifesting as urgency, cramps, or diarrhea. Gut irritants are more easily identified than intolerances because symptoms usually occur soon after eating the foods, are confined to the gut, and resolve fairly quickly. Dealing with gut

What should I do about COFFEE & CAFFEINE?

Caffeine has been proven as a performance enhancer in athletic circles. It used to be thought that coffee showed minimal benefits as compared to other forms of caffeine; in fact, early studies claimed other compounds present in coffee might actually be detrimental to performance.

More recent research has shown that caffeine in coffee matches caffeine from other sources. However, caffeine dosage depends on many factors, such as how the barista makes your coffee, what kind of beans are used, and how long the coffee is brewed.

Caffeine and coffee can have detrimental effects in the context of food intolerances, though. Caffeine generally increases gut motility, or the speed at which contents move through the gastrointestinal system. For those who are more sensitive to it, urgency, cramps, and diarrhea may occur. Because blood is being diverted away from the GI tract during exercise, the GI distress some athletes experience may be caused by a cup of joe—or their sports drink, gels, or bars that contain caffeine.

Both coffee and tea are also rich sources of salicylates. For athletes who are sensitive, headaches, flushing, and other symptoms can occur. If this is the case, as with all sensitivities to salicylates, amines, and/or glutamates, symptoms present not with initial exposure but once a threshold has been reached. With careful planning and avoidance of other trigger foods, sensitive individuals may still be able to reap the benefit of coffee or other caffeinated products without reaching the tipping point where symptoms emerge.

Of course, there are also studies identifying health risks, but it seems that on the whole, coffee in moderate amounts is healthy for the average person. If you already drink coffee, I don't necessarily recommend that you eliminate it unless you either suspect it is problematic or you try a base functional diet that includes coffee and continue to have symptoms.

Coffee has many other benefits beyond that of the sporting arena, including:[96]

Improved cognition and protection from dementia and Alzheimer's /
Rich source of antioxidants / Reduced risk of type 2 diabetes /
Potentially lower risk of stroke / Reduced risk of some types of cancers /
Protection against Parkinson's disease

irritants may simply be a matter of careful timing as opposed to avoidance. For instance, some people find that coffee poses no problems unless it is consumed just before exercise. Combining the effects of a gut irritant with the effects of exercise (a reduction of blood flow to the stomach and intestines) is more than enough to bring on GI distress. Keep a food diary to become aware of what you can and cannot tolerate and the quantities and timing of ingestion, especially in regard to exercise.

FOOD AVERSIONS

Food intolerance is primarily a physical or physiological reaction or response. However, it is impossible to uncouple the psychological effects of thoughts and beliefs, whether conscious or subconscious, and deny that they have an effect on how we view and tolerate foods. Even though a response may be all in the mind, there can be a very real physical reaction.

Food aversions are one instance where particular sets of circumstances or memories can turn you off a particular food for life, such as changing hormone levels in pregnancy or the association of a particular food with an event, person, or experience. Often, negative associations are the strongest, as with a harrowing food-poisoning episode or a stressful or anxiety-provoking event. When devising a nutrition plan for performance, any food aversions you have need to be taken into account.

It is often said that the mind is the difference between winning and losing. I think the mind decides whether we even start at all. This is not just true for elite athletes; it's true for everyone. Anxiety and lack of belief are performance crushers, whether you are worried about achieving the goal or task ahead or about how you will look in your workout clothes.

The power of psychology extends to food. We are so invested in food beyond its role as a fuel source: We connect to others through food, but we also connect memories, customs, and rituals to food—even in a sporting context. Many athletes have their favorite (or only) pre-competition meal that forms part of their pre-competition ritual. These habits and routines are calming, providing a sense of order and reliability even when nervousness takes hold. There is also a belief attached to these rituals, more so for some than others, that without a certain food or meal eaten at the correct time, they will have a bad performance. Conversely, there is good luck associated with foods: Having eaten them, individuals are buoyed with confidence.

Anxiety slows down gastric emptying, meaning you may be more sensitive to food aversions prior to competition.[97] The very thought of some foods can make your stomach turn, and this response can be enough to have a negative impact on performance. Don't try and push through food aversions; you will always be able to find something that you can tolerate well that will provide the nutrition you require for competitive demands.

Don't follow the advice in the sports magazine or copy someone else. Your approach needs to be individualized. If you have a rock solid belief that a steak the night before the game, meet, or race is going to give you the winning edge, then who am I to argue with you? The science might not be there to back up your claim and I could come up with an alternative that provides the recommended nutrition, but the advantages will pale in comparison to the power of belief.

EXERCISE-INDUCED ALLERGIES OR ANAPHYLAXIS

When the gut barrier is compromised as a result of exercise, food particles enter the bloodstream and trigger an immune response. This can occur with a food that is usually tolerated well. Crustaceans and wheat are the most common foods involved, but exercise-induced allergies or anaphylaxis can occur with any food. The key is that both the trigger food as well as exercise, most commonly high-intensity exercise, are needed to induce a reaction. In other words, if you were to eat that same food at rest, it would not cause any issues, and similarly, exercise would also be uneventful without eating that particular food. Extreme temperatures, humidity, and hormonal changes can also contribute to the reaction. As with other allergic reactions, symptoms include hives and itching, GI distress, as well as wheezing and difficulty breathing progressing to anaphylaxis. This condition is life threatening, but the food allergen does not typically need to be eliminated from the diet completely, rather avoided in the four to five hours prior to exercise.[98]

TESTING FOR FOOD INTOLERANCE

Celiac disease is one of the few food intolerances with a definitive test and diagnosis. A biopsy of the intestinal wall is taken to confirm the diagnosis. In other words, there is no gray area. When it comes to food intolerances, however, things are far less clear-cut. There are laboratories and clinics around the world that claim to be able to test for myriad food intolerances and sensitivities. Some of these use blood work, others use hair analysis or skin pricks, and some even use electrical conductivity and physical pressure. One of the strangest tests for gluten intolerance involves holding a piece of bread to the stomach and testing the arm's resistive strength with and without the piece of bread. Who wouldn't be skeptical of the validity of such a test? There are plenty of other tests available, none of which are proven, and some just as flawed as the bread test:

Blood testing. Despite the claim that blood testing detects food intolerances, this type of test is in fact looking for immunoglobulin G (IgG) antibodies. IgG antibodies are actually a marker of exposure to food proteins, not an indicator of allergy. So when blood testing comes back with a long list of foods that you are supposedly intolerant of, don't be surprised that all the foods you consume regularly and/or ate recently are on that list. Some research also indicates that presence of IgG antibodies may be a marker of food tolerance as opposed to intolerance. Different labs have returned different lists of food intolerances to the same people, and results from the same lab for the same person have also given different results.[99] In other words blood testing produces lots of false positives and false negatives and is not reliable or evidence based.

Hair analysis. While hair samples are reliable for testing in toxicology, there is no evidence that they can be used in detecting food intolerances.

Iridology. This test examines the iris of the eye for location and color of flecks, as well as any different textures, as proof of intolerance to particular foods. These tests do not pass scientific scrutiny.

Pulse testing or heart rate response. The subject eats different foods, and pulse rate is measured after each exposure. A rise is heart rate is said to indicate an intolerance. As any athlete knows from training with heart rate monitors, pulse is variable and subject to both conscious and subconscious changes, regardless of what is being eaten.

Electrical conductivity. Food extracts are introduced to an electrical circuit running between electrodes attached to two points of the body. Dips or interruptions in electrical charge are determined as being food intolerances. Results cannot be reproduced and show no difference between individuals with known allergies and intolerances and those without.

Strength testing. A food sample is either held in the hand or placed on the body, commonly under the tongue. Changes in muscle strength are said to reflect sensitivity to a given food. No scientific evidence supports this test.

Cytotoxic testing. Otherwise referred to as ALCAT tests, this procedure isolates white blood cells from blood samples and then combines them with different food extracts. A microscope is used to determine any movements or changes in the cells as an indication of a food sensitivity. These types of tests are unreliable and not reproducible.[100]

Breath analysis. This is the one method of testing that can reliably identify malabsorption of certain sugars or carbohydrates. When malabsorbed sugars reach the gut, they are fermented by bacteria and produce hydrogen or methane gas. Because some of this gas is absorbed through the intestinal wall and into the bloodstream, where it is eventually carried to the lungs, breath analysis can be used to detect the presence of these gases. This method can accurately identify lactose intolerance, where the milk sugar lactose is not broken down properly. An intolerance to fructose, sorbitol, glucose, and any combination of these sugars can also be tested for. Breath testing can also be used to diagnose small-intestinal bacterial overgrowth, in which higher than normal numbers of bacteria are present in the small intestine and can cause symptoms of pain, bloating, diarrhea, cramps—all symptoms that can also present with a food intolerance.[101] While breath testing might be an accurate method, it is quite expensive. Rather than pay to pinpoint a lactose intolerance, you could simply eliminate dairy from your diet and see what happens.

———

Other than breath analysis, currently none of the intolerance tests stand up to rigorous scientific scrutiny. However, huge advances are being made in this area, and hopefully one day there will be a scientific test that will help people reliably identify or quantify specific food intolerances and sensitivities. Somehow I doubt the bread to the stomach test will ever pass muster, but others do show more promise. Until that point, and perhaps even after, an elimination diet remains the gold standard in determining food intolerance and/or sensitivity. Foods contain complex chemicals and compounds that we have not even identified yet, let alone designed a test for, so even if a laboratory or medical professional says that you do not have any intolerances, if you feel better avoiding a particular food, then you should do so. It is easy to implement: it's noninvasive, it doesn't hurt, it's cheap, and you are in the driver's seat.

Consider the base functional diet an opportunity to conduct your own scientific research. Treat it like a scientific experiment—in other words, don't falsify data or cheat. Be confident in the process or you are likely to be swayed by others or blinded by your fears of giving up specific foods. I find that people often have a preconceived idea and then seek to validate it. Keep detailed notes throughout the process by tuning in to your body's signals and keeping an open mind. It's easy enough to find explanations to support your beliefs. For a true elimination diet to be successful and get to the root of the cause of any discomforts and symptoms, you must be ready to listen to your body and take note of what it has to say.

IDENTIFYING YOUR INTOLERANCES

Now that you're acquainted with the different food intolerances and sensitivities, it's time to figure out which ones are problematic for you. A base functional diet provides a structural framework for you to clean up your diet. The foods in the base functional diet have been selected because they are nutritionally dense, meeting your body's needs while simultaneously eliminating the most inflammatory foods. The most common irritants and allergens have been removed. Some widely prevalent foods high in FODMAPs and processed foods containing chemicals have also been removed so that total intake is likely to be below thresholds where they are well tolerated by the majority of people.

Not all of the eliminated foods are likely be an issue for you, but the base functional diet provides a nutritious starting point from which observations and identification of food intolerances can be more easily made. By simply removing inflammatory foods, most people see huge changes in health and performance. In other words, the symptoms you are experiencing may not be due to a food intolerance at all; instead, they are a reflection of how your body is trying to cope with a poor diet.

The base functional diet is simple enough so that you can easily note the effects of individual foods to help you decide whether they are problematic or not. Even so, not all foods in the base diet will be safe for everyone. If you know you are allergic to a food that is included in the diet, of course you will need to

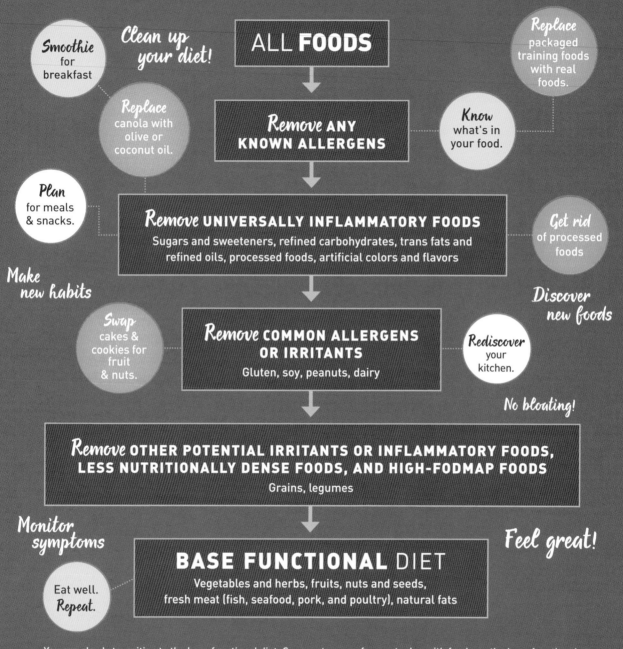

FIGURE 2. Getting to a base functional diet

Clean up your diet!

Smoothie for breakfast

Replace packaged training foods with real foods.

ALL **FOODS**

Replace canola with olive or coconut oil.

Remove **ANY KNOWN ALLERGENS**

Know what's in your food.

Make new habits

Plan for meals & snacks.

Remove **UNIVERSALLY INFLAMMATORY FOODS**
Sugars and sweeteners, refined carbohydrates, trans fats and refined oils, processed foods, artificial colors and flavors

Get rid of processed foods

Discover new foods

Swap cakes & cookies for fruit & nuts.

Remove **COMMON ALLERGENS OR IRRITANTS**
Gluten, soy, peanuts, dairy

Rediscover your kitchen.

No bloating!

Remove **OTHER POTENTIAL IRRITANTS OR INFLAMMATORY FOODS, LESS NUTRITIONALLY DENSE FOODS, AND HIGH-FODMAP FOODS**
Grains, legumes

Monitor symptoms

Feel great!

Eat well. Repeat.

BASE FUNCTIONAL DIET
Vegetables and herbs, fruits, nuts and seeds, fresh meat (fish, seafood, pork, and poultry), natural fats

You can slowly transition to the base functional diet. Swap out some of your staples with foods on the base functional diet list or change one meal at a time. Move on from here until your diet matches the base functional diet in terms of exclusions and inclusions. Keep in mind that the clock starts only when you reach this point, not when you begin making the smaller changes. This is important.

continue to eliminate that food as well. And allergies or intolerances to other foods in the base functional diet are still a possibility. However, with some detective work on your part, the simplicity of the diet will reveal hidden intolerances. From there, you can begin slowly and methodically reintroducing some healthy foods to your diet— including natural dairy foods and properly cooked and prepared legumes and whole grains. In the section on Eating for Performance (page 85), we will take a closer look at the macronutrients an athlete needs to maintain while following a base functional diet or any diet that accommodates food intolerances.

GETTING **STARTED**

It can be somewhat intimidating to stick to a diet that eliminates foods you eat regularly. If you are already making an effort to eat healthy, fresh foods, transitioning to a base functional diet really amounts to making some simple substitutions, being aware of what you are eating, and remaining committed to the goal. I believe most athletes fit into this category. For the athlete who relies on processed and packaged foods, it will be more difficult. However, by the same token these individuals will likely see the best results from making a change. Performing better in addition to looking good and feeling great is surely enough of an incentive to make you want to continue to eat the best foods you possibly can. The likelihood of improved health and vitality is an important bonus. You have nothing to lose by trying the base functional diet—it is chock-full of nutrients and almost a guaranteed step up from the majority of current diets.

Chances are good that you are coming to this program because you have some stubborn symptoms that you can't seem to shake. Before you begin a base functional diet, first rule out any medical cause for your symptoms. You are aware of the wide-ranging symptoms that accompany food intolerance that manifest themselves throughout the body's systems, and there will be plenty of crossover with other conditions. It is important that you not ignore the possibility that symptoms could be attributable to a serious underlying medical condition that requires diagnosis and treatment. Look to dietary causes only after determining there is no other known cause. An elimination diet like the base functional diet is really designed for people and athletes who are generally healthy but looking for improvements in performance and recovery.

If you suspect that celiac disease is a possibility but you are still eating gluten, get tested *before* eliminating foods containing gluten. For a definitive diagnosis, gluten must be present in the diet in a significant quantity or else you risk being misdiagnosed. Even minute exposure to gluten can be devastating for celiac sufferers, so it's important to know how vigilant you need to be. Precautions should be taken to avoid cross-contamination with foods that contain gluten—this includes shared kitchens and equipment, whether at home

Shopping list for the BASE FUNCTIONAL DIET

WHAT'S IN YOUR CART

- O Vegetables and herbs: All types (local, seasonal, organic if possible)
- O Fruits: All types (local, seasonal, organic if possible)
- O Eggs: Free range if possible
- O Poultry: Including turkey, chicken, duck, quail (free range, organic if possible)
- O Fish and other seafood: Wild caught
- O Meat: Including beef, lamb, pork, bison, venison (pasture raised if possible)
- O Nuts and seeds: All types
- O Coconuts: Fresh, milk, "butter"
- O Natural fats: Olive oil, avocados and avocado oil, coconut oil, nut oils

WHAT'S NOT IN YOUR CART

- O Sugars and sweeteners, including artificial sweeteners
- O Additives and preservatives (except salt)
- O Gluten grains and all other grains (including all foods made from grains: breads, pasta, cereals, bars)
- O Legumes (beans and lentils)
- O Soy and soy-based foods
- O Dairy and dairy-based foods
- O Foods for which you have known allergies or highly suspected intolerances
- O Vegetable oils (e.g., corn oil, soybean oil)
- O Trans fats and hydrogenated oils

or eating out. This is not the case for people with non-celiac gluten sensitivities.

It is vital that you be prepared. Try not to start the base functional diet if you know you have a stressful or busy week ahead. Withdrawal symptoms are likely, so you'll want to make things as easy as possible. If you suspect coffee or caffeine is an issue for you, it is preferable to reduce or eliminate it beforehand, as this withdrawal can be painful in its own right, making it hard to contemplate other changes or deal with other stress rationally. Stock up on foods that you can eat, and either put away or get rid of the foods you will be eliminating. Any elimination diet will be useless unless you

are vigilant and strict about totally avoiding specific suspected foods and components.

Get used to reading food labels and knowing any other terms that food manufacturers might use to disguise certain ingredients. In other words, if you are trying to determine if wheat is a trigger food for you, then you need to be aware of foods containing wheat starch as well as beer and other not-so-obvious sources of wheat. Without doing so, you are not truly testing your tolerance, and the true source of your symptoms and sensitivities will be harder to identify. Even trace amounts of the eliminated foods will undo all your efforts. The key is to focus on all the foods that you can eat.

Even if it feels as though this initial diet is very restrictive, there are still plenty of food choices, and I would encourage you to get excited about exploring all the possibilities. Heard of rambutan or celeriac? Try to break outside of your usual vegetables and fruits and explore the more exotic-sounding ones, or those that you think you don't like—even if you have never actually tried them or only tried them as a young child. Try a different cooking method, too. Often a vegetable that can best be described as "meh" when boiled or steamed becomes irresistible when roasted, that simple action allowing the natural sweetness and rich flavors to be drawn out.

I have included eggs and rice (and rice flour–based foods) in the base functional diet in an effort to make the experience a bit easier. I also find that both of these foods are especially beneficial to athletes when they are well tolerated. (If you suspect eggs may be an issue for you, see page 79.) Rice is a hypoallergenic food that is unlikely to be a cause of food intolerance for most people. For athletes in particular, rice can be a great source of easily digested carbohydrate and a good complement to a nutrient-rich diet. There aren't many nutrients in rice alone, so it is not meant to be a staple; it is accessible when eating out or traveling to races, and because it is low in fat and fiber, it makes a good pre-race meal.

Yes, this process does require you to cook more for yourself and also to take more responsibility for what you are eating. But really this is a small inconvenience when weighed against good health and improved performance. Cooking your own food has many rewards; not only is it easy to control and know exactly what you are eating,

but it also gives you invaluable insight into how foods are prepared, what they are likely to contain, and how to be more wary and conscious of suspect foods, preparations, and ingredients. A little knowledge is power when it comes to taking charge of your own health.

You don't need to become a gourmand or churn out restaurant-quality meals every day; in fact, the opposite is true. Keeping things simple is

How can you be sure you're getting your fill of nutrients?

You might be concerned that by eliminating whole grains you will miss out on fiber as well as nutrients and overall energy in the form of carbohydrates. Less than 10 percent of the general population eats the recommended five servings of vegetables each day—the average is reportedly a paltry 1.6 servings.[102] It is really hard to argue that a diet that is devoid of whole grains is unhealthy or nutritionally incomplete if those gaps are filled by vegetables, fruits, nuts, animal proteins, and good fats, all of which supply equal or even higher quantities of nutrients. The same can be said for both legumes and dairy foods. (The main concern in relation to avoiding dairy is calcium, which is addressed on pages 53–54.)

FIGURE 3. How to execute the base functional diet

Here is a look at how the process of identifying problematic foods plays out. This athlete was experiencing bloating, bathroom urgency, frequent headaches, and mood swings prior to starting the base functional diet. He had no other known allergies.

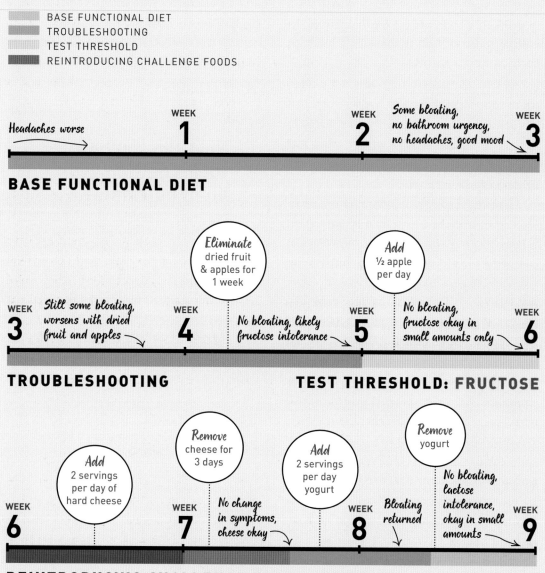

BASE FUNCTIONAL DIET
TROUBLESHOOTING
TEST THRESHOLD
REINTRODUCING CHALLENGE FOODS

Headaches worse →

WEEK **1**

WEEK **2**

Some bloating, no bathroom urgency, no headaches, good mood

WEEK **3**

BASE FUNCTIONAL DIET

WEEK **3**

Still some bloating, worsens with dried fruit and apples →

Eliminate dried fruit & apples for 1 week

WEEK **4**

No bloating, likely fructose intolerance →

Add ½ apple per day

WEEK **5**

No bloating, fructose okay in small amounts only →

WEEK **6**

TROUBLESHOOTING   TEST THRESHOLD: FRUCTOSE

WEEK **6**

Add 2 servings per day of hard cheese

WEEK **7**

Remove cheese for 3 days

No change in symptoms, cheese okay →

Add 2 servings per day yogurt

WEEK **8**

Bloating returned →

Remove yogurt

No bloating, lactose intolerance, okay in small amounts →

WEEK **9**

REINTRODUCING CHALLENGE FOODS: DAIRY

Next steps: This athlete could go on to test other challenge foods in the same way, noting symptoms.

one of the best ways to eat cleanly, and it's easy! Let a few quality ingredients speak for themselves. Having said that, you may also find yourself getting excited about getting in the kitchen, exploring new tastes, new foods, and new combinations. And that too is fantastic! You will find some of my favorite recipes on pages 111–204 to get you started on the base functional diet.

It's also a good idea to involve your family, roommates, or friends as much as possible in your shopping, cooking, and eating adventures. People, including and especially kids, are more likely to be excited about what they are eating (particularly if it is unfamiliar or anything green) if they have also been involved in choosing the produce and preparing the meal. Changing your eating habits and sticking to dietary goals is much easier if you have the whole house on board. To simplify things further, I will share some of my tricks to help you manage your time spent shopping and cooking so that maintaining healthy habits can become second nature for you.

STEP 1: ADOPT A BASE FUNCTIONAL DIET

Three weeks is really the minimum amount of time required because it can take this long for withdrawals to subside and trace elements of suspect foods to diminish.[103] The three-week trial should also include a week of no symptoms. So if you start the base functional diet and your symptoms resolve immediately, then stick with it for three weeks. The same goes if your symptoms resolve after one to two weeks. If symptoms lift at three weeks, then follow the diet for another week, making it four weeks total. If at four weeks you still have symptoms, it's time to reevaluate what other foods might be problematic (see Step 2).

When your symptoms decrease, you will know the program is working. Don't be surprised, however, if symptoms get worse for the first few days. Withdrawal symptoms are pretty common, but if they are severe you can consider modifying the initial elimination phase. First eliminate the foods that you find easy to avoid and simply cut back on the foods that are causing the withdrawal. Over the course of one or two weeks, work toward fully eliminating the most difficult foods. Once you've achieved this, start the three-week base functional diet phase.

Once all of your symptoms are gone (for a full week) and you are feeling good, continue to Step 3, where you'll begin reintroduction of some foods.

KEEP A FOOD DIARY

Keep a food diary over the course of your base functional diet to monitor symptoms as well as energy and mood. It is also important to consider other factors such as work stress, emotional situations, financial concerns, disrupted sleep, travel, training, illness—any number of which can influence how you feel. These notes are vital to the process and will show if there is a pattern developing

You might find that your symptoms on the base functional diet either have nothing to do with your gut or that while you may have GI issues, there are other symptoms present as well. If you experience sensitivity to light or scents (laundry detergents, perfumes), headaches, or mood changes, this may indicate a sensitivity to natural food chemicals such as amines, glutamates, and salicylates, which need to be identified, eliminated, and retested. Other common complaints attributed to food chemicals could extend to skin irritations, any part of the GI system (from mouth to anus and including complaints such as diarrhea or constipation), urinary system problems, respiratory issues such as wheezing and coughing, muscle and joint pain, and poor sleep and recovery.

If you continue to struggle with frequent symptoms even after considering sources of FODMAPs and/or food chemicals, or if you are worried or confused about food choices, menu ideas, or nutrient intake, it might be worthwhile to consult with a nutritionist or dietitian for individual support. This can be a tricky area of intolerance to navigate alone.

PROTOCOL FOR TESTING FODMAPS

Review the examples of foods high in FODMAPs (page 55) to identify the foods that might be giving you trouble, and eliminate these foods or groupings of foods from your diet.

Once your symptoms are relieved for at least a week (and this may take as long as six to eight weeks to occur), then you can begin testing the groupings of food by carbohydrate types one at a time to determine your tolerance level. You might find that particular types of carbohydrates are more or less tolerated than others. It also doesn't mean that you cannot have any of the "problem" foods, merely that you will find an amount that keeps you symptom-free. Anything over that amount will tip you over your personal threshold, eliciting symptoms.

Keep in mind that this is not an exhaustive list, so you might want to check on individual foods not included. A research team at Monash University has developed online resources and an app to help navigate high- and low-FODMAP food items. Because testing of foods for FODMAPs continues, the resources are continually updated at www.med.monash.edu/cecs/gastro/fodmap.

PROTOCOL FOR TESTING FOOD CHEMICALS

1 Identify and eliminate the foods high in natural chemicals (see page 61). Avoid all of these foods for a minimum of three weeks, or however long it takes to get to five to seven consecutive symptom-free days. If symptoms persist, seek help from a nutritionist.

(During this time, don't forget to consider other sources of chemical exposure that might be causing or adding to your reactions: cleaning agents, garden sprays, shampoos, soaps, etc.)

2 Include at least three servings of foods from either the salicylates or amines groups below. Eat these foods every day for seven days while avoiding foods from the alternative list. It's necessary to restrict yourself to the test foods as some foods are high in both salicylates and amines, so they won't be helpful in determining which chemical you have a sensitivity to. Because glutamates are found in foods that also contain amines, there is no need to test these separately.

Salicylate test foods. Apples, asparagus, capsicum, carrot, cinnamon, cucumber, curry powder, mango, nectarines or peaches, strawberries, watermelon.

Amine test foods. Cocoa, dark chocolate, or ripe bananas.

3 If you do not react to the test foods, that group can be safely included in your diet after the testing phase is over.

If you do react, remove the foods, wait at least a week, and then try testing each food individually, again ensuring you eat the food every day. This will help you determine your own tolerance threshold: Carefully document your intake—both timing and amount—so that if a reaction occurs, you know how much you can eat over how many days before the threshold is breached. Even if there is not a reaction initially, eating more of these foods can cause a buildup of chemicals to the point where symptoms recur.

Remember, reactions can occur immediately, the next day, or several days later. Also, for more-sensitive people it can take days, weeks, or even months for residual levels of built-up chemicals to subside to a symptom-free level. This can cloud and complicate identification and testing of foods.

4 Repeat steps 2 and 3 with the other group of test foods.

Because this can be a long, tricky process, I recommend that you work with a nutritionist if you are struggling. This will ensure you aren't eliminating too many foods over a lengthy period and risking potential deficiencies.

STEP 3: REINTRODUCE FOODS

This step is really a series of small steps and again relies on your investigative powers to monitor and evaluate the effects of each food as you reintroduce them one at a time. There is no set order for reintroduction. It might depend on what you suspect you are intolerant of, what you feel you miss the most, or what would make a significant difference to your enjoyment or ease of cooking and shopping. Remember, the goal is to maintain a diet that is free of most inflammatory foods. So that donut or toaster pastry, while convenient and perhaps something that you miss, is not the type of food to reintroduce to your diet.

Food challenges allow you to confirm that a food is problematic if your symptoms reappear (sometimes more strongly than before) when it is added back in. Some foods will require a more nuanced approach. If you at first notice symptoms, you might try adjusting the quantity of the food consumed to find your tolerance level. In some cases, you might find you are okay eating a small amount or that timing is critical. For example, some people can tolerate small amounts of cheese or yogurt, but eating them closer to a training workout or in larger amounts will induce symptoms. Do not reintroduce any foods that cause an allergic reaction or that you have been medically advised to avoid (e.g., if you have celiac disease, do not test gluten as a challenge food). If you feel best when you are eating only the foods on the base functional diet, then feel free to stick to these foods. There is no nutritional necessity to add additional foods if you don't feel better doing so.

DAIRY

Test each type of dairy individually. Dairy intolerance can be caused by a number of factors, and this approach will determine what and how much you can eat. Is the issue the lactose or the casein? Can you tolerate fermented dairy foods? Butter? Goat's milk? (Goat casein is more similar to human casein than cow's milk is, so some people tolerate this dairy better.) Do you find that you react to cheese but not to other dairy foods? If so, then it is likely the natural amines present in the cheese are a problem for you rather than lactose. It makes sense to try to figure out what you are reacting to so that you can still enjoy and benefit from the nutrients present in well-tolerated dairy foods. (Note: If you do have celiac disease, then you are more likely to not tolerate casein, the other major protein aside from lactose in dairy products.)

GRAINS & LEGUMES

Test grains one at a time. Remember, some individuals are sensitive to gluten, others may be sensitive to gluten-like proteins (or other proteins) in grains. The only way to see how you react is by testing each type one at a time. Keep in mind that the goal is not to end up with a diet that is high in grains, thereby reducing your intake of other more nutritious foods (such as vegetables). *Do not reintroduce refined grain products.*

PROTOCOL FOR A FOOD CHALLENGE

1 Pick a food to reincorporate into your diet and eat this food at least twice a day for seven days. Stop if symptoms recur before seven days. This indicates a strong reaction; consider this food an intolerance and move onto the next challenge food.

2 If symptoms do not recur during the seven days, remove the food and revert to the base functional diet for three to four days. This provides a good perspective to see how you feel with and without that food. Continue to take notes and monitor throughout.

3 If you decide there is no change in symptoms, this food can be added to your list of tolerated foods.

Repeat the process with other foods.

The same advice holds true for introduction of legumes. Test each type and determine which and how much of a certain type you might be able to tolerate. When it comes to grains and legumes, even if they are well tolerated, keep in mind that they should complement other elements of a healthy (base functional) diet as opposed to becoming staple foods. Also keep in mind that these foods are best tolerated and more easily digested when prepared properly in the slow traditional manner, including soaking and cooking thoroughly.

STEP 4: REPEAT AS NEEDED

Because food intolerances/sensitivities can change over time or present in different ways, you can always tinker with your diet to find what works best for you to make you feel good. The idea is to be aware of what you are eating and how you are feeling and adjust things as necessary. If it is obvious what foods you are reacting to, you can try eliminating just them. If it is hard to pinpoint the cause, then you can do a more restrictive elimination experiment again, testing foods carefully as you reintroduce them. You might also find that foods you once reacted to are no longer a problem (again, excluding allergies).

EATING FOR PERFORMANCE

It's entirely possible to successfully train and race while you are on a base functional diet. In fact, for some people a base functional diet might be the long-term solution. Dietary restrictions can raise a lot of questions for athletes because sports nutrition guidelines tend to champion a mix of traditional carbohydrates, lean protein, and low-fat foods. Let's take a closer look at how you can get the macronutrients you need as an athlete while also managing your food intolerances.

CARBOHYDRATES ARE VITAL TO PERFORMANCE

There is debate raging in the popular and scientific worlds over carbohydrates. For those who are overweight, diagnosed with diabetes, or at risk for developing diabetes, a lower carbohydrate diet is well substantiated.[104] However, the best research continues to back the notion that adequate carbs are essential for optimal sports performance. The amount of carbs required differ depending on whether you compete in a power-based sport, a technical sport, or an endurance sport, but carbohydrates play an important role.[105]

FOODS HIGH IN CARBOHYDRATES

Bread, cereals, cakes, and cookies might all be off the table, but there are still plenty of high-carbohydrate foods to enjoy. The main sources include:

Fruit. All fruits are great sources of carbs. Apart from avocados, they are all devoid of both fat and protein, so essentially they are pure carbohydrate.

Root vegetables and squash. Sweet potatoes, yams, carrots, parsnips, celeriac, pumpkin, and various types of winter squash all provide carbs.

Rice and rice-based products. These can be used to provide a more highly concentrated source of energy, whether as a pre-race meal or to meet higher energy demands, without the bulk or fiber of other carb sources. If you are focused on weight loss it is better to minimize reliance on these products.

As a reference, all of these foods contain 50 g of carbohydrates:
11 dried apricots, 2 medium bananas, 2½ cups fruit salad, 2 cups grapes, 12 cups strawberries, 1 large potato, 2½ cups sweet potato, 14 cups green beans, 6 thick rice cakes (or 10 thin ones), 1 cup cooked rice, 1¼ cups rice noodles, 3 Tbsp. honey

During digestion, the body breaks down carbohydrates into glucose, which is stored in the muscles and liver as glycogen. During exercise, this glycogen is converted back to glucose and is used for fuel to power activity. The amount stored is typically enough to power workouts of around 90 minutes before fat stores are mobilized for energy or additional carbohydrates are needed.

Carbohydrate intake is one of the biggest concerns for endurance athletes. Eliminating breads, cereals, and pastas leaves a significant void that will need to be filled. But there are other ways to meet carbohydrate recommendations. Wheat and grain products can provide plenty of energy, but as we have seen they may also cause intolerances or lead to nutrient-poor choices. Many athletes need to seek out more nutrients to help their bodies cope with training stress. A platform of general health allows athletes to train hard and recover well. What's more, if you are eating a high-quality diet based on your best foods, you can better adapt to your training loads, which ultimately means you become fitter and faster.

HOW MUCH & WHEN?

The ideal amount of carbohydrate will fuel your daily workouts optimally without adding excess energy that could promote weight gain. There's some nuance to defining what that amount is for you and how it should change to reflect the demands of your training (duration, intensity, and frequency) as well as your season goals and optimal body composition. Table 8 outlines current daily carbohydrate recommendations based on training intensity and volume. This is merely a guide; your individual target will vary depending on your goals for a particular day or where you are in the season. For instance, while the table recommends a high-carbohydrate intake for an athlete following four hours of strenuous training, it is unlikely that this same athlete will need to eat this much day in and day out. Carbohydrate intake can take place either before, during, or after exercise. However, post-exercise intake is the most important because it allows the body to replenish glycogen, which aids recovery and tops off energy stores in preparation for the next workout.

If you are trying to reduce your body weight, less refined (mostly these will be grain-free) sources of carbohydrates increase the volume of food consumed with fewer total calories and more nutrients. In other words, to reach 50 grams of carbohydrates, you'll need to consume foods such as fruits and vegetables, in higher quantities, for example 2½ cups of sweet potatoes. This is in contrast to refined grain sources; a single bread roll could contain 50 grams of carbs. It is easy to see which would be more filling and which might be easy to over shoot in terms of quantity.

TABLE 8. Daily carbohydrate targets for athletes

INTENSITY / DESCRIPTION OF TRAINING	CARBOHYDRATE (per kg)
Light *Low-intensity or skill-based activities*	3–5
Moderate *Moderate exercise, about 1 hour/day*	5–7
High *Moderate to high-intensity exercise, 1–3 hours/day*	6–10
Very high *Moderate to high-intensity exercise, 4–5 hours/day or more*	8–12

Source: Adapted from IOC Consensus statement: http://www.olympic.org/documents/reports/en/en_report_833.pdf, © IOC

There are times when energy needs are high but more compact forms of carbohydrates work better. This is especially true during or immediately before races. More refined foods, including sugars and natural sweeteners, in limited amounts can play a role in athletic fueling and are generally well tolerated. You can see how to incorporate

Curb your carbs with vegetables

Non-root vegetables also contain carbohydrates; however leafy greens, zucchini, and broccoli are also high in either water content and/or fiber, so they are comparatively lower in carbohydrates. Use this to your advantage if you are looking to lose weight. These vegetables also offer an easy way to reduce your daily carbohydrate intake when training volume or intensity is less demanding.

these foods in the sample menu in Figure 5. Further guidelines are provided in A Smart Approach to Sports Foods, pages 98–101.

Even in short races or competitions lasting less than one hour, small amounts of carbohydrates or just mouth rinses with a glucose-containing sports drink stimulate the central nervous system and improve performance. It is evident that these performance benefits are not due to the extra energy provided, since it takes time (around 30 minutes) for ingested sugars/carbs to reach the bloodstream and be delivered to working muscles. This contrasts to efforts of 1–2.5 hours, where a range of 30–60 g/hour carbohydrate is a good target, and for longer events, where consuming up to 90 g/hour may be beneficial and provide the energy needed to sustain maximal efforts. These targets depend on various factors including body size, fitness level, pre-race consumption, and individual tolerance.

FIGURE 5. Sample menu including refined carbohydrates

Here is a sample menu for a 155 lb. (70 kg) male athlete in hard training (up to three hours per day) that provides 515 g of carbohydrate (CHO), which equates to approximately 7.5 g CHO/kg.

Pre-workout breakfast: 50 g CHO
Leftover roasted potato, 1½ cups:
   50 g CHO
2 eggs: 0g CHO

During workout: 80 g CHO
Fruit & Nut Bars (p. 192): 80 g CHO

Post-workout breakfast: 75 g CHO
Blueberries, 1 cup: 20 g CHO
Coconut Apple Cinnamon Pancakes, 2
   (p. 128): 30 g CHO
Honey, 1 Tbsp.: 18 g CHO
Almonds, 1 handful (¼ cup): 7g CHO

Lunch: 65 g CHO
Baked sweet potato, 1 large: 36 g CHO
Cooked kale or spinach, 2 cups: 15 g CHO
Salmon, 1 fillet: 0 g CHO
Nectarine, 1 small: 14 g CHO

Snack pre-workout: 80 g CHO
Chocolate Cherry Coconut Recovery Bites, 2
   (p. 194): 80 g CHO

Dinner: 130 g CHO
White rice, 2 cups: 90 g CHO
Mixed vegetables (e.g., broccoli, carrots,
   cauliflower, peas), 2 cups: 40 g CHO
Steak, small fillet: 0 g CHO

Dessert: 35 g CHO
Baked Banana Split, 1 serving (p. 176):
   35 g CHO

TABLE 9. Timing carbohydrates for training & racing

TIMING / PURPOSE	TIME FRAME / DURATION	AMOUNT
PRIOR TO TRAINING AND RACING		
General fueling up	Less than 90 min.	7–12 g/kg^{-1} per 24 hr. as for daily fuel needs
Pre-event fueling (pre-race meal)	More than 60 min.	1–4 g/kg^{-1} consumed 1–4 hr. before exercise
	Less than 60 min.	No specific requirements
Carbohydrate loading	Preparation for events with more than 90 min. of sustained/intermittent exercise	24–48 hr. of 9–12 g/kg^{-1} body mass per 24 hr.
DURING WORKOUT		
Brief exercise	Under 45 min.	Not needed
Sustained high-intensity exercise	45–75 min.	Small amounts, including mouth rinse
Endurance exercise including "stop and start" sports	1.0–2.5 hr.	30–60 g/hr.
Ultra-endurance exercise	Over 2.5–3.0 hr.	Up to 90 g/hr.
BETWEEN SHORT RACES OR HARD TRAINING EFFORTS		
Speedy refueling	Less than 8-hr. recovery between two races or very hard workouts	1.0–1.2 g/kg/hr. for the first 4 hr., then resume normal daily fueling

Source: Adapted from IOC Consensus statement: http://www.olympic.org/documents/reports/en/en_report_833.pdf, © IOC

WHAT IS CARBO-LOADING?

There is good evidence to support carbo-loading for events lasting longer than 90–120 minutes (depending on individual circumstances).[106] This means that you do not need to carbo-load for your local 5K (or any 5K), sprint triathlon, or criterium race. If you are racing an Ironman or running a marathon, then smart carbo-loading practices are warranted. In all the excitement around race day, it's easy to get carbo-loading wrong. Here are a few of the mistakes you'll want to avoid:

> Processed carbohydrates loaded with sugar—cookies and ice cream
> Buffet and pasta parties (even if they are included in the race registration)
> Ditching all good eating habits and practices
> Increasing caloric intake above normal

As training tapers off before a big event, your energy demands will be reduced, which means that you are carbo-loading by eating the same amount. Furthermore, if you have a history of gastrointestinal problems on race day, you will want to reduce your intake of proteins and fats, which increases the ratio of carbohydrates in your diet.

In preparation for race day, you might find that more refined, less fibrous foods are easier to digest. The following options work well for most people and could all be included on the base functional diet:

> Rice
> Rice noodles
> Sports foods (see page 98) as tolerated, or other sugar-based foods and products
> Honey or other sweeteners (if fructose is tolerated)
> Fruit (possibly peeled, canned, and/or cooked to reduce fiber content)

Research supports the idea that carbohydrate-rich diets are essential for optimizing recovery and assisting the immune function of athletes who train and compete at a high intensity on a regular basis. The rationale is that the body produces cortisol as a stress response to high-intensity exercise, but cortisol production is dampened by the intake of glucose (carbohydrates). Put simply, carbohydrates appear to be important in maintaining hormone balance and immunity, especially in hard-training athletes.

However, there still are benefits to training in a carbohydrate-depleted state and forcing the body to become more efficient at using fat stores as fuel. You can essentially achieve these adaptations by training early in the morning before breakfast or by doing a second session in the afternoon after a hard workout in the morning. This teaches your body to tap into crucial fat stores without compromising recovery. It also allows you to go into key workouts optimally fueled so you can push yourself to your limit and maximize training adaptations.

FAT PLAYS A CRUCIAL ROLE

Athletes have long avoided fat as a result of traditional health and sports nutrition guidelines, but we need to think about both the quantity as well as the quality of fat in our diets. Within the body, fat is an essential part of the structure and function of each and every cell. In addition to playing an important role in immunity, hormone production and delivery, and vitamin absorption, fat is also an important source of fuel.

Even in the leanest of individuals, fat is used as a source of energy. In theory, each of us has enough body fat to fuel us for days on end without being in danger of running short. However, glucose is clearly the body's preferred fuel source for high-intensity activity, and it is in short supply. Only about 500 grams of glycogen is stored in the muscles and liver, and this can be blown through pretty quickly—in about 90 minutes of lower-intensity exercise and less time for higher-intensity efforts. This is why recommendations for carbohydrate intake during exercise begin with sessions lasting longer than 60–90 minutes.

There is emerging evidence to suggest that fat adaptation might be an effective performance strategy for endurance athletes, particularly for ultra-endurance athletes competing at very low intensity over extended time periods.[107] In theory, fat could provide a better source of energy for these athletes, eliminating the need for on-course nutrition and the GI distress associated with it, preventing energy crashes so effort can be sustained for very long periods of time. There have also been promising anecdotal reports to support the practice, especially among the ultra-endurance world, although the actual scientific evidence remains somewhat limited. Most scientific studies are not supportive of this approach for the majority of athletes. Their findings show that while high-fat, low-carb diets can increase fat-burning as the body's primary fuel, this is a result of down-regulating glycogen use. In other words, the lower carbohydrate diets encouraged increased fat utilization for energy, but perhaps only because the subjects became less efficient at using glycogen sources. No performance gains were seen, and long-term studies are as yet lacking. It will be interesting to see the developments in this space over coming years.

It is often the case that laboratory or controlled scientific findings lag behind what athletes are experiencing in the field. Again, your personal experimentation is what counts because everyone has to find their ideal place on the spectrum of macronutrient ratios. What works best for race day may differ from your day-to-day macronutrient intakes for general health and well-being. The key message from the latest research is that you shouldn't be afraid of including plenty of healthy fats in your diet. The recipes in this book certainly reflect this thinking.

HEALTHY FATS FOR YOUR DIET

Olive oil

Avocados

Grass-fed butter and other full-fat dairy

Nuts

Coconut oil, macadamia oil, walnut oil, other nut oils

Fatty fish, especially salmon, sardines, and mackerel

Fats in grass-fed or wild-caught meats

In addition to playing an important role in immunity, hormone production and delivery, and vitamin absorption, fat is also an important SOURCE OF FUEL.

WHY ATHLETES NEED PROTEIN

Holding a coveted position among the macronutrients, protein is (almost) never cast as the nutrition villain. There are fat-haters and carb-cutters who pin the blame for rising rates of obesity and ill health on one or both of those macronutrients, but protein has mostly evaded the negative press. It has maintained an aura of importance in the general population as a nutrient essential for supreme health, an attitude that is perhaps even more prevalent in the athletic world. Protein is essential, but just how much to eat, when to consume it, and what are the best sources remain subjects of confusion and misplaced notions.

Protein is critical to the human body, playing an important role in both structure and function. It is found in muscle, bone, skin, hair, and virtually every other body tissue. Protein also makes up the enzymes necessary for many chemical reactions and metabolic processes, as well as the hemoglobin that carries oxygen in your blood. Protein deficiencies are devastating, and although rare in the Western world, in areas of poverty the result of this type of malnutrition can result in stunted growth, loss of muscle mass, compromised immunity, weakening of the heart and respiratory systems, and ultimately, death.

Protein is also important for healthy aging, and adequate intake is essential for helping to maintain muscle mass. Muscle mass into the later stages in life is of interest to the aging athlete who wants to continue biking, running, or throwing down weights in the gym, but it is also key to living an active life, maintaining independence, and preventing falls. Around age 30, the body begins to gradually lose muscle. Strength training and good nutrition that includes adequate protein is the best approach to maintaining the muscle mass that your sport requires and attenuating some of the natural losses that occur with aging.[108]

GOOD SOURCES OF PROTEIN

Chicken breast, 3½ oz. (100 g): **28 g**
White fish, 1 fillet: **22 g**
Mussels, 12: **20 g**
Beef, 4 oz. (100 g): **27 g**

Non-meat options
Hard-boiled egg, 1: **7 g**
Almonds, 1 oz. (25 g): **4 g**
Peas, 1 cup (145 g): **4 g**
Hemp protein powder, 20 g (2 Tbsp.): **8 g**
Chia seeds, 20 g (2 Tbsp.): **4 g**
Flax seeds, 20 g (2 Tbsp.): **4 g**

Dairy foods, if tolerated
Hard cheese, 1 oz. (30 g): **6 g**
Yogurt, 1 cup (200 g): **12 g**

Legumes, if tolerated
Garbanzo, pinto, kidney, or black beans,
 1 cup (165 g) cooked: **13–15 g**

Grains, if tolerated
Quinoa,1 cup (185 g) cooked: **8 g**

HOW MUCH & WHAT TYPES?

Some amino acids are made within our bodies, either manufactured from scratch or made by modifying other amino acids. Those known as the essential amino acids need to come from food. Animal sources of protein contain all the different types of essential amino acids (see Table 10), whereas plant sources lack one or more and hence foods must be carefully combined to provide the complete spectrum.

As an athlete, you need more protein than someone who has a sedentary lifestyle. In Table 11 you can see how both volume and intensity of physical activity create more demand for protein. If you are not getting enough protein in your diet, it may mean that the body will opt to break down muscle mass in order to supply the body with essential amino acids. Furthermore, your ability to adapt to increased training loads will plummet, along with athletic performance.[109]

In terms of sports performance, the timing of your protein intake is perhaps even more important than getting enough protein. Research shows that eating foods containing protein throughout the day in all meals and snacks is most effective for building or maintaining muscle and adapting to training.

Athletes are well aware that the 30 minutes following exercise will make or break recovery, especially when training programs demand multiple workouts in a day. Protein intake in this time frame has long been a priority because it increases muscle protein synthesis rates. Eating protein before or during exercise is also an effective way to inhibit muscle breakdown and stimulate synthesis or muscle protein. Although it does not improve the performance of that effort, it may help with recovery and consequently promote training adaptations, indirectly contributing to performance gains. Eating protein prior to going to bed at night has also been shown to stimulate muscle growth and repair, support adaptation to training, and prevent muscle breakdown.

The protein recommendations for athletes can be summarized with three main points:[110]

> Get 20–25 grams of protein with each main meal, including a pre-bedtime snack.
> Fit in 20–25 grams of protein immediately in the first 30–40 minutes after training.
> If workouts are longer than 2–3 hours, also include some protein in your fueling prior to and during the workout.

TABLE 10. Amino acids

ESSENTIAL AMINO ACIDS	NON-ESSENTIAL AMINO ACIDS
Isoleucine	Alanine
Leucine	Arginine
Lysine	Asparagine
Methionine	Aspartic acid
Phenylalinine	Cystine
Threonine	Glutamic acid
Tryptophan	Glutamine
Valine	Glycine
	Histadine
	Hydroxyproline
	Hydroxyglycine
	Proline
	Serine
	Taurine
	Tyrosine

TABLE 11. Estimated protein requirements for athletes

GROUP	PROTEIN INTAKE (g/kg/day)
MALE ATHLETES	
Elite endurance athletes	1.6
Moderate-intensity endurance athletes*	1.2
Recreational endurance athletes[†]	1.0–1.2
Intermittent sports (e.g., soccer, basketball, martial arts)	1.4–1.7
Resistance/strength athletes	1.6–2.0
FEMALE ATHLETES	
Elite endurance athletes	1.4
Moderate-intensity endurance athletes*	1.0
Recreational endurance athletes[†]	0.8–1.0
Intermittent sports	1.2–1.4
Resistance/strength athletes	1.4–1.7
SEDENTARY MEN AND WOMEN	0.8–1.0

* Exercising approximately four to five times per week for 45–60 min;[†] Exercising four to five times per week for 30 min. at < 55% VO_{2peak}

Source: B. Campbell et al. "International Society of Sports Nutrition Position Stand: Protein and Exercise." *J Int Soc Sports Nutr* 4 (2007): 8, doi:10.1186/1550-2783-4-8.

CAN YOU HAVE TOO MUCH?

It is very easy, even for a strength-based athlete with the highest requirements, to hit the upper end of protein requirements without specifically focusing on large amounts of protein at each meal (see list of protein sources for how quickly protein adds up). But can you have too much? Studies have shown that when protein exceeds around 2g/kg/day, the calcium excreted in the urine is increased. Based on these observations, some researchers have warned that these calcium losses might be putting athletes (and non-athletes) at increased risk of bone loss or weakened bones and fractures. However, these concerns have since been put to rest with subsequent research that shows while increased protein intake did initially lead to more calcium being excreted, over the longer term this trend was reversed and indeed higher protein intakes were associated with stronger bones and decreased rates of osteopenia (bone loss).[111] Other concerns in regard to protein intake have centered on kidney function and health. Again, the bottom line is that for healthy individuals getting more than 2g/kg/day, there is not a health risk. If you suffer from kidney function disorders, then certainly intake must be restricted. Consult your doctor about how much protein you should consume if you're concerned.

High-protein diets (where protein supplies around 30 percent of total energy) have long been popular for weight loss, and there is plenty of evidence to support their effectiveness.[112] For athletes, high-protein diets can also be effective in helping to achieve body fat and weight goals by helping to maintain muscle mass in calorie-restricted weight loss diets. In other words, for athletes interested in weight loss, it is vital that protein be an important part of their diet or weight loss could be a result of muscle wastage, in which case strength and endurance is lost, undermining performance.

MULTIVITAMINS & SUPPLEMENTS

When it comes to nutrition and how it affects different interactions and functions in the body, we still know very little. We also know relatively little about food and nutrients. We know there are carbohydrates, proteins, and fats, and we have identified various vitamins and minerals as well as other compounds. However, phytonutrients cover a broad range of compounds for which we have very little information. Phytonutrients are the components of fresh fruits and vegetables that make eating whole, real foods much more effective than any supplement or pill. Multivitamins and supplements are limited by what we have discovered and isolated and what we can best replicate in a laboratory. Furthermore, because the nutrients in a multivitamin are delivered all at once, utilization is compromised as a result of the interactions between individual nutrients. In other words, some nutrients block or boost the absorption of others.

Research also suggests that supplemental antioxidants could reduce the training adaptations and health gains of exercise.[113] It has long been known that exercise produces free radicals. At one time we thought it would be beneficial to reduce these free radicals by taking antioxidant supplements, which would ostensibly help both recovery and the ability to cope with training loads while also maintaining health and immunity. But it is now accepted that these free radicals may actually be essential to achieving some of the health benefits of exercise, stimulating adaptation so we can get fitter and faster. It seems that the large doses of antioxidants found in supplement form suppress these important adaptations. By contrast, when smaller quantities of antioxidants are consumed as part of a whole-food diet, this is not the case. It's yet another example of how the benefits of a nutrient-rich diet cannot be achieved by shortcuts and pills. In other words, eat your fruits and vegetables.

Research also continues to build in the area of sports-specific supplementation. There are some promising results emerging, along with plenty of results of limited, questionable, or even dangerous use. But the fact remains that even those supplements that are proven to be beneficial to performance offer very marginal gains. The biggest advantage will always come from what you eat and how you train day in and day out. Promises made from supplement manufacturers are meaningless unless you have a good framework in place. Don't be distracted by the thing that could deliver a 0.5 percent improvement and lose sight of everything else that makes up the other 99.5 percent.

hunger signals and follow your intuition—this method is proven to be reliable in the long run. Once you have removed unhealthy foods and foods you don't tolerate from your diet, portions and timing can become a more natural part of an athletic lifestyle. Be smart about fueling, but take the time to enjoy the food you eat.

EATING WELL
FOR LIFE

I really want you to enjoy your food. Even if you find you are best served by avoiding or limiting certain foods, there should never be a sense of deprivation or resentment about what is on (or off) your plate. The goal is to discover and incorporate foods that you enjoy eating that also fit your intolerances and sensitivities. At first, like any change to routine or habit, these shifts in diet and lifestyle might seem difficult. However, they should become easier both with time and with the positive reinforcements that come with results. Be kind to yourself. You are allowed and even expected to make mistakes. You are allowed and expected to stray on occasion from what you know to be ideal. But the goals of improved health and performance remain the same, and overall dietary patterns and habits are what ultimately matter. The following section provides some information to help keep you on track and assist with removing some of the barriers that come with changes, including those of financial, social, and time management pressures.

Regardless of what your intolerances and sensitivities are, eating for health and performance will likely entail some changes to your lifestyle. Eating healthy foods, the kind that fight inflammation and promote overall health, means you will spend more money on high-quality foods and more time preparing your own foods. It's my hope that through this process you will rediscover your love for food and that will give you plenty of incentive to adapt food to your lifestyle. In the meantime, I'll share with you some of my own strategies.

How to **SAVE MONEY** on healthy foods

There is no denying that the cost of buying fresh produce is greater than filling your cart with packaged foods. The expense is easier to justify if you keep in mind the long-term costs related to health care as well as the non-financial costs of not functioning and achieving to your potential. There are clever ways, however, in which you can keep costs down:

Keep an herb garden. Growing a few of your favorite herbs in pots will add some natural nutrients to your diet and help you save some money at the market. Just snip off what you need each day.

Plan meals around produce that is in season.

Buy grocery items in bulk when you see a good price and cook some, freeze some, store some.

Don't be afraid of using "imperfect" produce. Rain blight or a small bruise doesn't mean the taste will be compromised.

Buy the less-popular cuts of meat and poultry. Instead of chicken breast and beef fillets, buy a whole chicken or beef ribs or stew meat.

If you have access to a market or delivery service, buy your meats directly from the farmer.

Join a co-op or sign up for a CSA (community-supported agriculture) share for fresh, locally grown seasonal produce.

Use every part of your produce. Don't throw the broccoli stalks or the beet leaves on the compost heap—they are both edible and delicious.

Don't spend money on supplements! There is no evidence to support their effectiveness; in fact, they may even be harmful. It's always better to eat your nutrients.

Invest in storage containers to reduce spoilage. Many households throw out more food than they eat. Make things stay fresh a little longer by storing them properly.

Practice cooking. With some basic skills you can cook from what you have on hand rather than having to buy new ingredients for every recipe.

Never throw out meat bones. Use them to make your own stock.

Don't buy salad dressing. It's much cheaper to make your own. Simply mix oil, vinegar, seasoning, and add herbs or spices, if desired.

TIME-SAVING TIPS *to get you into the kitchen*

Cooking for yourself can take a little more time. Don't be intimidated by the commitment or the possibility of making a mistake—just find a recipe to inspire you and get into the kitchen. Cook in bulk whenever you can and store or freeze the unused portions. Leftovers always make good meals and are convenient, too.

When traveling or really pressed for time, buy pre-chopped vegetables. While they are more expensive, if it makes the difference between cooking and eating well or eating processed foods, it's worth it.

Keep things simple. You might enjoy getting in the kitchen and cooking up a storm, but not every meal needs to be culinary wizardry. You can't go wrong with basics like trays of roasted root vegetables, steamed greens, and a steak or fillet of fish.

Take your time. Slow-cooking can be the best way to save time in the kitchen. Throw a roast in the oven with a little seasoning, and let the oven do all the work. Several hours later, the smell of a delicious dinner will be wafting through your warm house without requiring much effort from you.

Prep ahead in your spare time. If you know you have a busy week ahead, spending a little time in the kitchen on the weekend can pay dividends. Simply chopping, sorting, and storing some vegetables can make a huge difference.

Cook with what you have and learn a little about ingredients and how to cook and combine them. This helps with planning as well as minimizing last-minute shopping runs for extra ingredients.

Plan ahead. For some people, having a menu planned for the week works really well. I have to admit I am not one of these people, but I know others who find that this level of organization helps them not only keep on track but also save time throughout the week.

Share the task of cooking with friends and family. Swapping dishes can be fun and save time for both families.

How to **STAY THE COURSE**
on the base functional diet and beyond

Life is full of surprises and challenges, so sticking to new habits can be tough. Accepting that things won't always be easy is the first step, but it helps to have a plan for when things start to feel too hard—whether it's the daily pressure of time management or having to defend your dietary choices to friends and family. The following list will help get you started, but add your own tips and tricks as you identify your own hurdles along the way.

Have snacks and quick meal options readily available. Chopped veggies stored in airtight containers, hard-boiled eggs, trail mix, avocados, fresh fruit, or leftovers. When hunger strikes fast and furious, you will be less tempted to resort to other options if you have healthy food and snacks on hand.

Try not to associate deprivation with the foods you are intolerant of. Tell yourself that of course you can eat it if you want, you just don't want to eat it because it gives you migraines, or flares up your eczema, or hurts your stomach. If it helps, keep written reminders of all your symptoms on the fridge.

Let go of trying to be perfect. It's human nature to fail or fall short. If you expect perfection, you are setting yourself up to fail. Instead, focus on improving and try to be better each day or with each meal. Sounds kind of like a training plan, doesn't it?

Treats/cheats. Chocolate has a role to play in health, with cocoa being one the richest known sources of polyphenols (antioxidants). Chocolate, albeit dark chocolate that has not been overly sweetened, along with coffee and red wine have also been shown to be beneficial in improving and maintaining healthy gut flora. All of these foods, though, can cause reactions in some individuals, likely due to the naturally occurring food chemicals they contain or the caffeine in coffee acting as a gut irritant to increase motility. If you are able to tolerate these foods, they can be reintroduced. Having these foods, which confer health benefits yet can also be viewed as treats, can be really helpful in sticking to more restrictive diets. If you look forward to a small square of dark chocolate to finish the day, that can help you avoid other less-healthy temptations.

When eating out or with others, stick up for yourself. Don't let peer pressure be your undoing. If you are unsure of what's in your food or on the menu, be sure to ask.

Other tips for a lifestyle of HEALTHY EATING

Being conscious of what you are eating is part of becoming connected to your food and its origins. However involved you can be in the process—from growing to preparing and cooking—you will develop a greater appreciation for food. Learn how to savor different flavors, and you will enjoy greater variety in what you eat. Most important, food provides so much more than fuel; eating is a social activity that connects and unifies us.

Sit down to eat. Avoid eating in the car or on the run, or at least don't make it a daily habit. I know it might sound difficult, but even taking five minutes to sit and enjoy lunch can be revitalizing.

Try never to eat alone. Food is social, and eating in a group can help you stick to good resolutions. Surround yourself with healthy people, and you will eat better. Or conversely, you can be the role model.

Get the whole family involved. This doesn't mean that everyone has to avoid foods just because one person has a food intolerance, but eating healthily and avoiding inflammatory foods as much as possible is something that everyone will benefit from.

Don't eat at your computer or desk, and never eat in front of the TV. It can be really tempting to think you need to save time or maybe just unwind, but mindless eating is never a good idea.

Avoid attaching negative emotions to food. Stop thinking about food in terms of guilt and instead think about food in terms of quality nutrition and enjoyment. Focus on how the food makes you feel as opposed to emotional eating, which only results in feeling bad.

Eat foods you like. Yes, there will be foods you like that are now restricted, but that doesn't mean you have to eat foods you don't enjoy. If you happen to hate broccoli, choose something else instead.

Eating healthy foods, the kind that FIGHT INFLAMMATION and promote overall health, means you will spend more money on high-quality foods and more time preparing your own foods.

RECIPES FOR THE BASE FUNCTIONAL DIET

THESE RECIPES exclude gluten, grains (except rice), soy, legumes, dairy, additives, and preservatives. If you have additional allergies or food intolerances, also eliminate those foods as part of your base functional diet. Gradually reintroduce quality foods to determine what additional foods you can tolerate.

BREAKFAST

FRITTATA *with butternut squash & basil*

SERVES **6**

Everyone needs a few staple meals to turn to when short on inspiration. If you can make a simple frittata, you will never go hungry! It's easy to prepare and versatile enough to be served as breakfast, lunch, or dinner. Serve hot out of the oven, at room temperature, or straight from the fridge. Sub in your own favorite ingredients or seasonal offerings to make this dish your own.

2 Tbsp. coconut oil, melted and divided
4 cups (560 g) butternut squash,
   peeled and cubed
1 red onion, sliced
3 cups (90 g) baby spinach
1 cup (135 g) frozen peas
Sea salt and pepper
12 eggs, lightly beaten
Generous handful fresh basil leaves, torn

Preheat the oven to 350°F (180°C).

In a large bowl, drizzle 1 tablespoon oil over the squash. Toss to coat, then roast the squash on a rimmed baking sheet until it's tender and starting to turn golden, about 40–45 minutes. Set aside to cool.

Preheat the oven broiler to medium-high.

Warm a large, oven-safe skillet over medium heat. Add the remaining 1 tablespoon oil and the onion, and sauté until translucent. Add the baby spinach, peas, and roasted butternut squash pieces. Stir to wilt the spinach and warm through. Season with salt and pepper to taste.

Pour in the beaten eggs and gently shake the pan so that the eggs and vegetables are evenly distributed. Cook until the edges start to set. Place the pan in the oven and cook until puffed and golden, about 5–10 minutes. Remove from the oven and top with the torn basil leaves. Let sit for 5–10 minutes before serving.

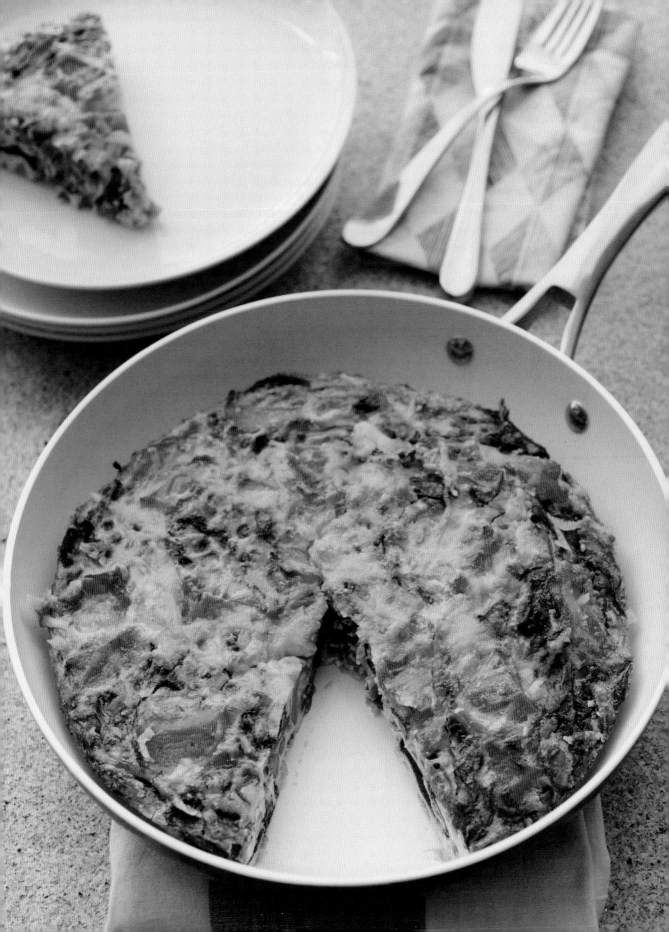

SWEET POTATO
HASH BROWNS *with poached eggs*

SERVES 4

Make this for a weekend breakfast or on a morning when you have a little more time. If you end up with leftovers, the hash browns are still tasty the next day.

1 lb. (450 g) sweet potatoes, peeled
1 medium onion, grated
2 eggs, lightly beaten
1 Tbsp. fresh parsley or chives, chopped
Sea salt and pepper
2 Tbsp. coconut oil, divided

POACHED EGGS

2 tsp. white vinegar
4 eggs

Preheat the oven to 250°F (130°C).

Grate the sweet potatoes into a colander. Use your hands to squeeze out as much moisture from the grated potatoes as possible (this will prevent the hash browns from being mushy). Squeeze them again inside a few paper towels, then transfer the sweet potatoes to a large bowl. Add the grated onion, the lightly beaten eggs, and parsley or chives and mix well. Season with salt and pepper to taste. Divide the mixture into 8 equal portions and shape into round patties.

Heat half of the coconut oil in a large skillet set over medium heat. When it is hot and shimmering but not smoking, add 3 or 4 hash brown patties. Press down on them with a spatula until they are about 1 inch (2.5 cm) thick. Fry until golden brown, about 2–3 minutes, then flip and fry another 2–3 minutes. Transfer the cooked hash browns to an oven-safe dish and keep them warm in the oven while cooking the remaining hash browns in the rest of the coconut oil.

To poach eggs: Fill a large saucepan a little over half full with water, add the vinegar, and set over medium heat until almost simmering—the water will have tiny bubbles rising from the bottom of the pan. Use a spoon to stir the water to create a whirlpool effect (this helps keep the egg intact). Crack an egg and place it gently into the center of the whirlpool, opening the egg as close to the water as possible. Turn off the heat, cover, and let cook without stirring for 2–3 minutes for a soft yolk and 3–4 minutes for a more solid yolk. Remove the egg with a slotted spoon and drain on a paper towel. You can cook the eggs one at a time using this method or all at once without stirring.

Place two hash brown patties on each plate and top with one poached egg. Serve immediately.

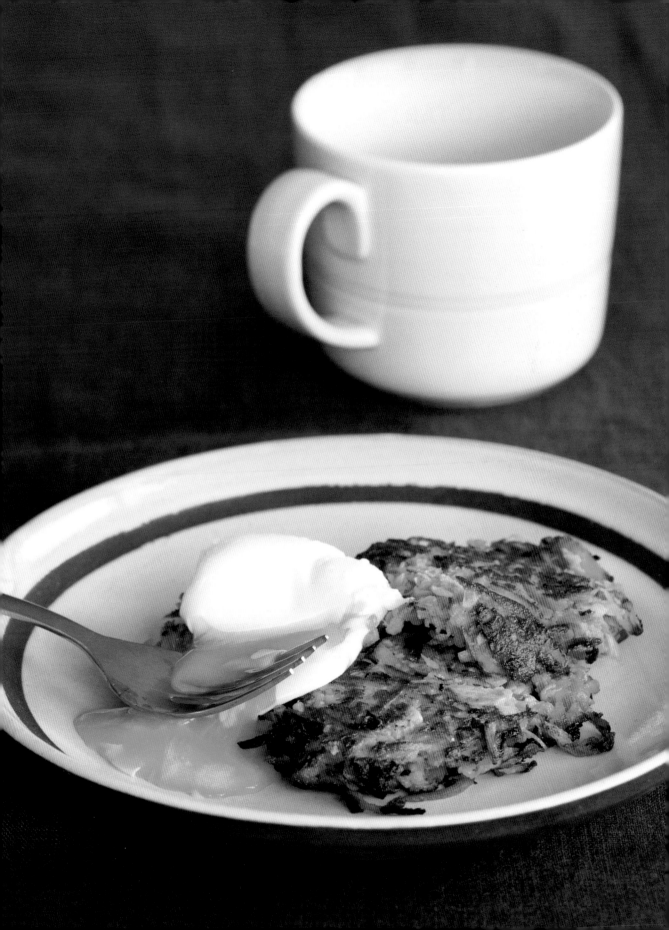

BACON EGG TARTS

SERVES 6

Heavy on protein and fat but light on carbs, bacon egg tarts are a good rest-day option. They can also be a post-workout snack if you have replenished carbs during your workout. When I have friends over for brunch on the weekend, I put out a spread that includes these tarts.

6 slices bacon
6 eggs
Sea salt and pepper
1½ Tbsp. fresh thyme, chopped
   (or other fresh herb of choice,
   e.g., dill, chives, or parsley)
3 Tbsp. scallions, chopped

Preheat the oven to 400°F (200°C). Grease 6 cups of a standard nonstick muffin tin with coconut oil.

Cook the bacon in a skillet until cooked but not browned. Drain on paper towels.

Line the sides of the muffin tin cups with the pieces of bacon, creating a ring. Carefully crack an egg into the center of each ring, season with salt and pepper to taste, and bake in the oven until the egg whites are set, about 15 minutes.

Remove and let cool for 3–5 minutes. Sprinkle with the herbs and scallions and serve with some wilted spinach or a small green salad.

Makes 6 tarts.

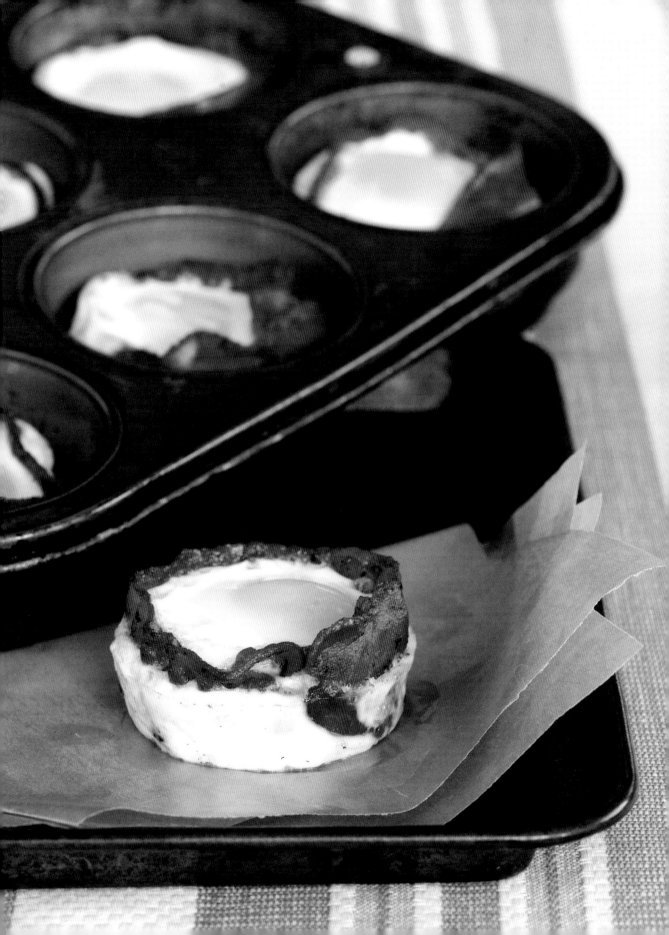

BAKED SAUSAGE CAPONATA

SERVES 4

This dish does take a little time, but the oven will do the bulk of the work. Caponata can be cooked in advance and simply reheated in the oven for 10 minutes while the sausages are cooking. Lots of sausages have gluten, wheat, and other preservatives and flavors, so look for sausages that are nitrate and filler free at farmers markets and local butchers.

1 large eggplant
1 bell pepper, cored and seeded
2 zucchinis
4 tomatoes, each cut into 8 wedges
2 Tbsp. olive oil
1 sprig fresh rosemary, chopped,
   stem removed
Sea salt and pepper
4 raw sausages (about 3 oz. each)
2 Tbsp. fresh parsley, roughly chopped

Preheat the oven to 350°F (180°C).

Chop the eggplant, bell pepper, and zucchini into 1-inch (2.5-cm) pieces and place on a large rimmed baking sheet with the tomato wedges. Drizzle with the olive oil and toss to coat. Sprinkle the rosemary over the vegetables and season with salt and pepper to taste. Place the sausages on top of the vegetables and bake for 30–40 minutes.

Turn over the sausages and return to the oven for another 20–30 minutes or until they are golden and the vegetables are cooked down, rich and sticky. Sprinkle with the parsley and serve.

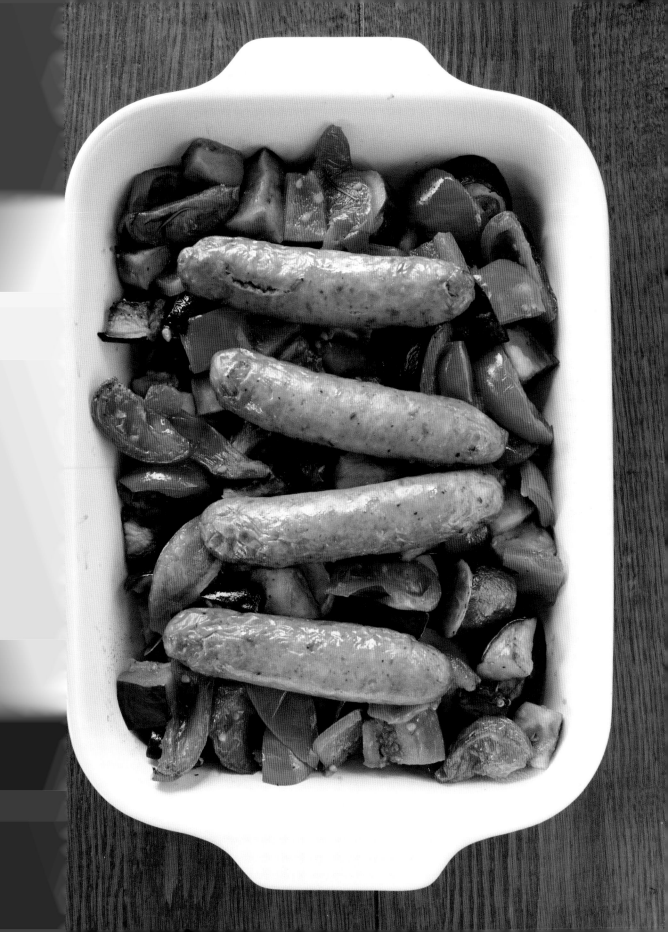

BANANA CINNAMON BREAD

SERVES 5

When I make banana bread, I use different flour combinations to allow for different intolerances or allergies. This variation uses coconut flour, which gives the bread nice flavor and a lot of fiber. I also use plenty of cinnamon; if you want a subtler flavor, use just 1 teaspoon. Change up the add-ins—use dried fruit for naturally sweeter bread or use nuts to add texture and a bit more fat and protein. For a real treat, try adding dark chocolate chips.

Scant ½ cup (50 g) coconut flour
1 tsp. gluten-free baking powder
1 Tbsp. cinnamon
Pinch of sea salt
¼ cup (30 g) unsweetened dried cranberries, raisins, or chopped walnuts
2 large (or 3 medium) very ripe bananas
5 large eggs (or 6 small ones)
1 tsp. vanilla extract
¼ cup (60 ml) coconut oil, melted

Preheat the oven to 350°F (180°C). Line a 4×8–inch (1 L) loaf tin with parchment paper.

Combine the coconut flour, baking powder, cinnamon, salt, and dried fruit or nuts in a medium-sized bowl. In a separate bowl mash the bananas, then add the eggs and whisk to combine. Stir in the vanilla and coconut oil. Add the wet ingredients to the dry ingredients and mix well.

Pour the batter into the prepared loaf tin and bake for 30–40 minutes. Remove from the oven when the loaf is golden on top and a skewer or toothpick inserted into the middle of the loaf comes out clean. Let rest for 5–10 minutes before slicing and serving.

Makes 10 generous slices.

BANANA BLUEBERRY BREAD

SERVES 6

¾ cup (120 g) rice flour
¼ cup (40 g) potato flour
¼ cup (30 g) tapioca flour
¼ cup (25 g) almond flour
2 tsp. gluten-free baking powder
1–2 tsp. cinnamon
3 large bananas
⅓ cup (80 ml) coconut oil, melted
½ cup (120 ml) coconut cream or almond milk
1 tsp. vanilla extract
2 eggs
¾ cup (115 g) frozen blueberries

Preheat the oven to 350°F (180°C). Line a 4×8–inch (1 L) loaf tin with parchment paper.

Mix together the flours, baking powder, and cinnamon in a large bowl. In a separate bowl mash the bananas and mix in the coconut oil, coconut cream or almond milk, and vanilla. Add the banana mixture to the flour mixture and stir thoroughly until combined.

Beat the eggs until thick and creamy—you are aiming to incorporate lots of air to help the loaf rise. Add half the beaten eggs to the batter and stir gently until combined. Add the other half and stir until just mixed. Gently stir in the frozen blueberries.

Pour the batter into the prepared loaf tin and bake until the loaf is golden on top and a skewer or toothpick inserted into the middle of the loaf comes out clean, about 60–70 minutes. Let rest for 5–10 minutes before slicing and serving.

Makes 12 generous slices.

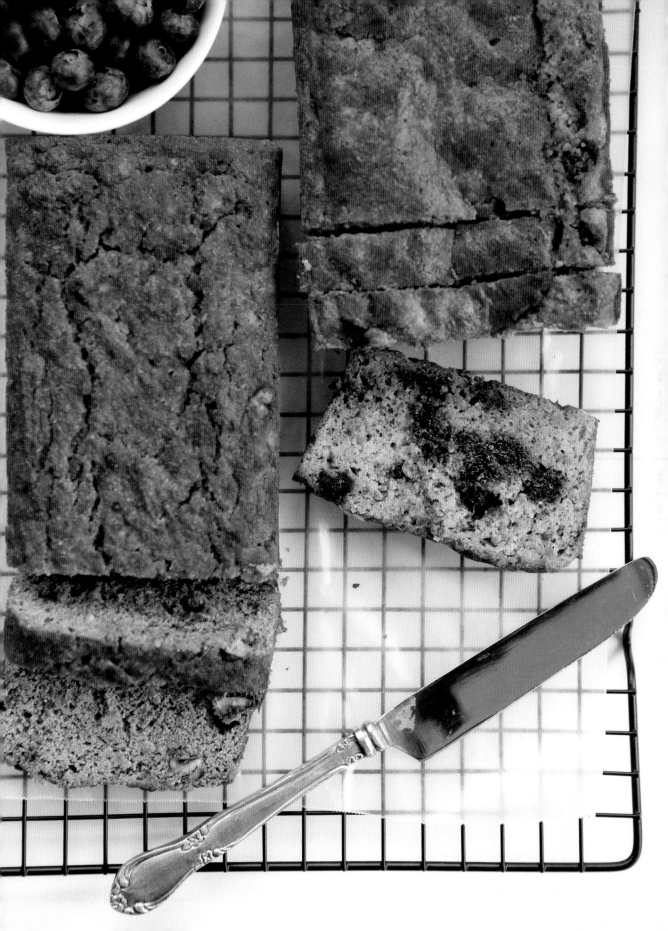

RICE PORRIDGE *with orange, pistachio & mint*

This porridge keeps well for a few days in the fridge. It is a nice option for a pre-race meal because it is also delicious served cold, like rice pudding.

½ cup (100 g) short-grain rice (such as arborio)
1 cup (240 ml) coconut milk or almond milk
1½ cups (350 ml) water
Juice and zest of 1 orange
1 Tbsp. almond butter
1 Tbsp. pistachios, shelled
1 Tbsp. fresh mint leaves, finely chopped

Rinse the rice well in cold water before placing it in a large saucepan. Add the milk, water, orange juice and zest and cook over medium-low heat, stirring often until the liquid is absorbed and the rice is cooked through, about 20 minutes.

Remove from heat and stir in the almond butter. Serve topped with the pistachios and mint leaves and extra coconut milk, if desired.

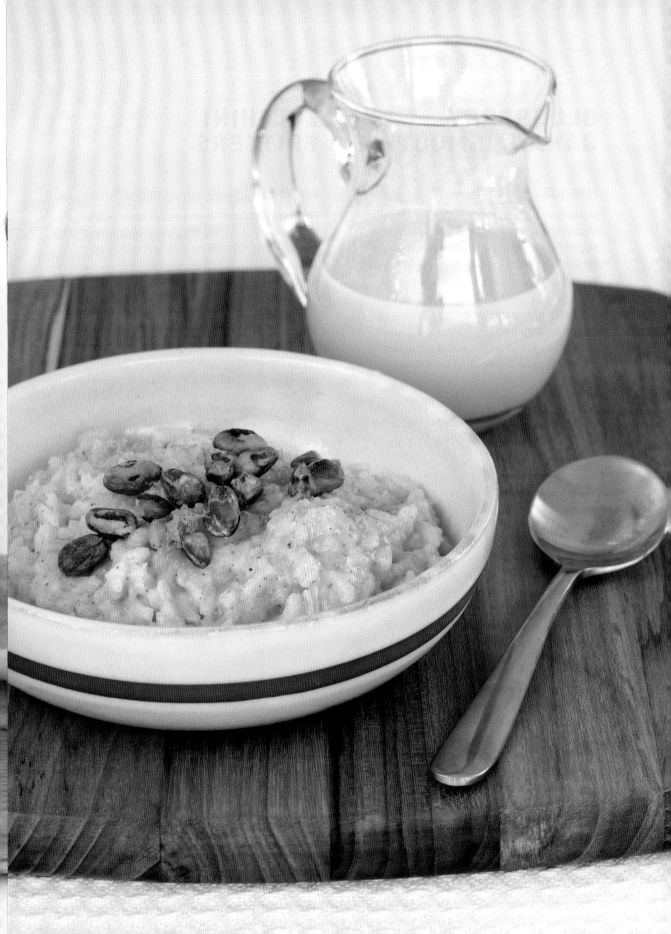

Coconut APPLE CINNAMON PANCAKES

SERVES 4

Everyone needs a sweet treat every once in a while, particularly after a long run or a hard gym workout. These pancakes are just decadent enough while still being surprisingly healthy. Serve them to your skeptical family members or friends, who will be quickly converted.

1 medium apple, peeled and cored
½ cup (60 g) tapioca flour
½ cup (80 g) rice flour
1 tsp. cinnamon
1 egg, lightly beaten
½ cup (120 ml) water
1 Tbsp. coconut oil
1 cup (140 g) fresh berries
1–2 Tbsp. coconut cream
1 Tbsp. shredded coconut, unsweetened

Preheat the oven to 250°F (130°C).

Cut the apple into large chunks, place in a small saucepan, and cover with water. Bring to boil and simmer gently until very soft, about 10–15 minutes. (Alternatively, place the apple pieces in a microwave-safe bowl with ½ cup (120 ml) water. Microwave on high for 2 minutes.) Cool, then mash thoroughly or puree.

Combine the flours and cinnamon in a large bowl. In a separate bowl combine the apple puree, egg, and water and mix well. Add the wet ingredients to the dry ingredients and mix thoroughly.

Heat the coconut oil in a skillet set over medium heat. Drop ¼-cup dollops of the batter into the pan. Cook until the edges start to set and small bubbles appear in the batter. Flip and cook for another 1–2 minutes or until cooked through and lightly browned on each side. Transfer the cooked pancakes to an oven-safe plate and keep them warm in the oven (or, alternatively, cover with foil) while cooking the remainder of the pancake batter.

Top with fresh berries, a little coconut cream, and some shredded coconut.

Makes 8 pancakes.

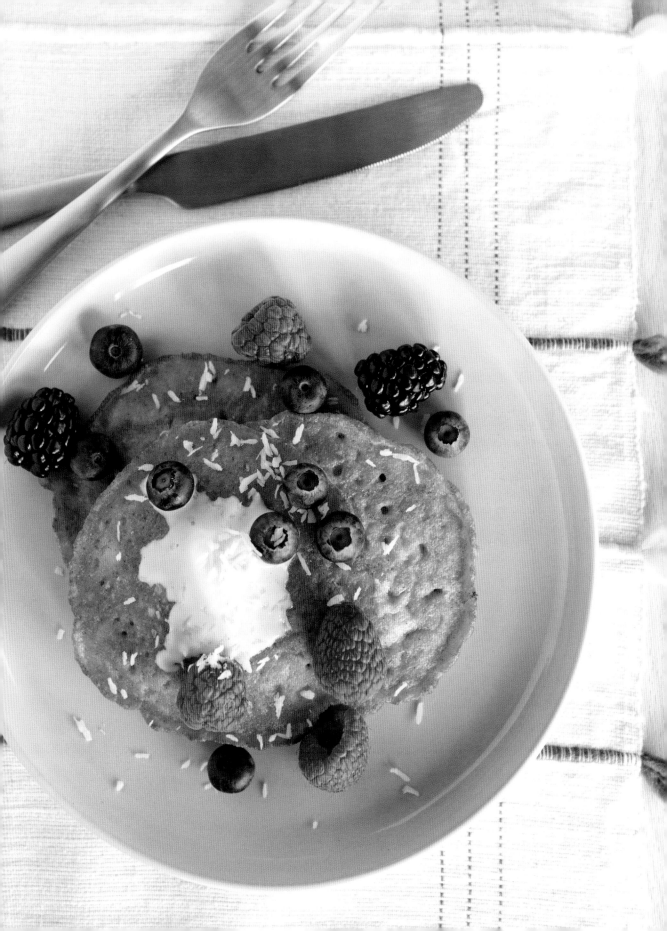

APPLE SAUSAGE
BREAKFAST BURGERS *with grilled tomatoes*

SERVES 4

These "brekky" burgers help fill the hunger gap between an early breakfast and dinner. You can also make and freeze the cooked sausage patties ahead of time to make for faster breakfasts.

8 lettuce cups (large whole leaves of
    romaine or iceberg lettuce)
2 Tbsp. coconut oil, divided
½ medium onion, finely chopped
1 clove garlic, crushed
1 apple, cored and grated
1 tsp. dried sage
1 Tbsp. fresh parsley, chopped
2 tsp. fresh chives, finely chopped
1 lb. (450 g) ground pork or turkey
Sea salt and pepper
2 tomatoes, sliced
½ cup (120 g) sliced avocado or guacamole*

* Optional; see recipe on page 138.

Carefully wash and dry the lettuce leaves, keeping them intact, and set aside.

Heat half the coconut oil in a large skillet set over medium heat. Sauté the onion, garlic, and grated apple until the onion is translucent and the apple is soft. Transfer to a food processor, add the herbs, and pulse until finely chopped but not pureed.

In a large bowl combine the ground pork or turkey, the apple and herb mixture, and salt and pepper and mix well. (It's easiest to use your hands to do this.) Shape into 8 patties.

Add the remaining tablespoon of oil to the skillet and heat over medium. Add the patties, cooking for about 4 minutes per side until cooked through. Remove and drain on paper towels. Add the sliced tomato to the pan and grill for 1–2 minutes per side until browned.

Place the lettuce cups on serving plates, top with a patty, grilled tomato, and avocado or guacamole (if using).

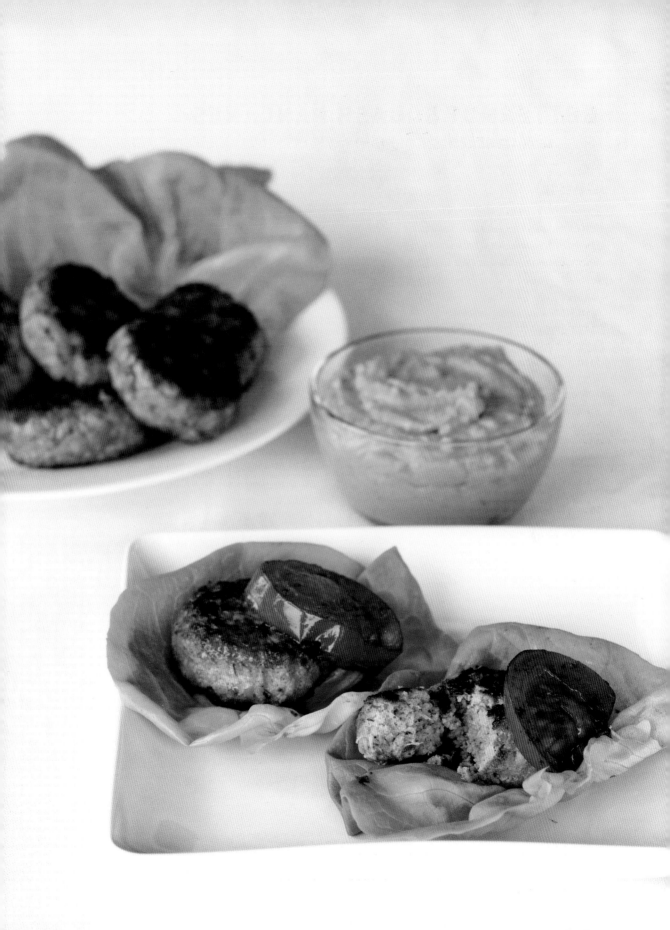

BUTTERNUT SQUASH PANCAKES
with smoked salmon

SERVES **2**

If you have cooked leftover butternut squash, this is a quick and easy way to transform it, or you can begin with raw squash. These mini pancakes pack way more nutrients than the regular flour-based ones, and paired with the avocado and smoked salmon, they make a decadent and satisfying breakfast. They could also be served cold as canapés with your choice of topping.

1 cup (240 g) cooked butternut squash, mashed or pureed, or 2 cups (280 g) peeled and cubed raw butternut squash
2 eggs
1 Tbsp. coconut flour
½ tsp. gluten-free baking powder
2 Tbsp. coconut oil, divided
4 slices smoked salmon
1 avocado, sliced

Preheat the oven to 250°F (130°C).

If you are using raw squash, place it into a microwave-safe bowl. Cover with water and microwave on high until very soft, about 6–8 minutes. Drain, then mash using a fork or puree with a hand blender.

Mix together squash, eggs, coconut flour, and baking powder until smooth.

Heat 1 tablespoon of the coconut oil in a skillet set over medium-high heat. Add half the batter in spoonfuls and cook, turning as the edges start to set. Turn and cook for another minute until lightly golden and cooked through. Transfer the cooked pancakes to an oven-safe plate and keep them warm in the oven (or, alternatively, cover with foil) while cooking the remainder of the pancake batter. Add the rest of the oil to the pan and repeat with the remaining batter.

Serve the pancakes in stacks of 4–5 per plate with slices of smoked salmon and sliced avocado.

Makes 8–10 mini pancakes.

COCONUT FLOUR is very high in fiber and very dry, meaning that it needs to be used sparingly and with lots of other wet ingredients such as eggs or oil, or in this case, pureed squash. One tablespoon of flour might seem like a small amount, but add any more and your pancakes will be dry and crumbly.

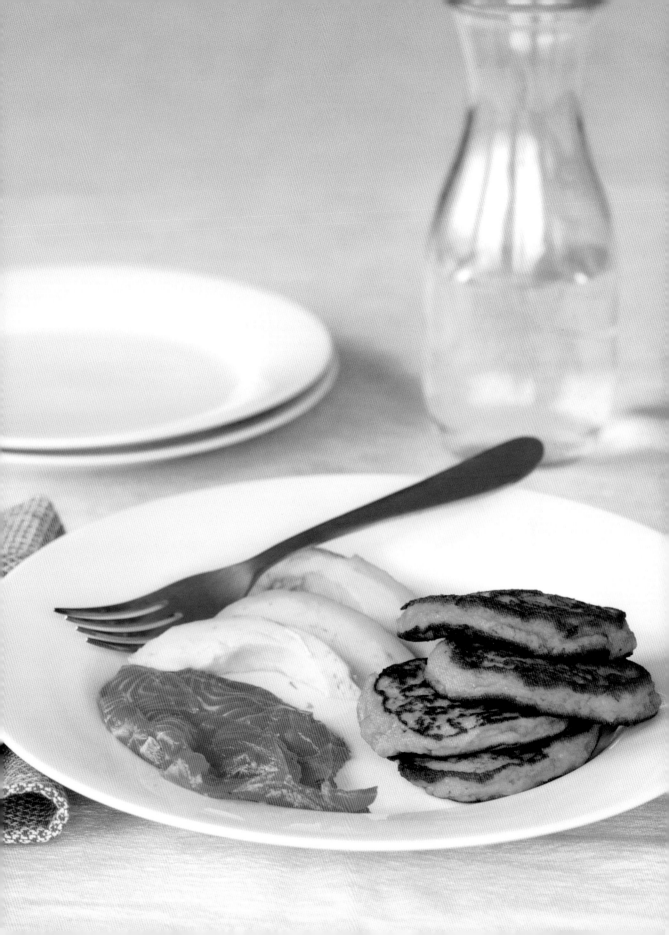

FRUIT & NUT GRANOLA

SERVES `6-8`

For those times when you want a more traditional breakfast option, this granola is good to have on hand. Pack some small portions to eat as trail mix or in place of packaged bars.

2 cups (240 g) walnuts, chopped
1 cup (145 g) almonds, chopped
1 cup (65 g) pumpkin seeds
1 cup (90 g) shredded coconut, unsweetened
2 Tbsp. coconut oil, melted
1 cup (120 g) dried cranberries, unsweetened, or other fruit

Preheat the oven to 300°F (150°C).

Combine the nuts, seeds, and coconut in a large bowl. Add the coconut oil and toss well to combine. Pour the mixture onto a large, ungreased rimmed baking sheet and spread in a thin layer.

Bake until golden brown, about 20–25 minutes. Add the dried fruit and stir.

Serve while still warm with almond or coconut milk and fresh fruit. Cool completely before storing. Granola will keep in an airtight container for about 10 days.

Makes 6 cups.

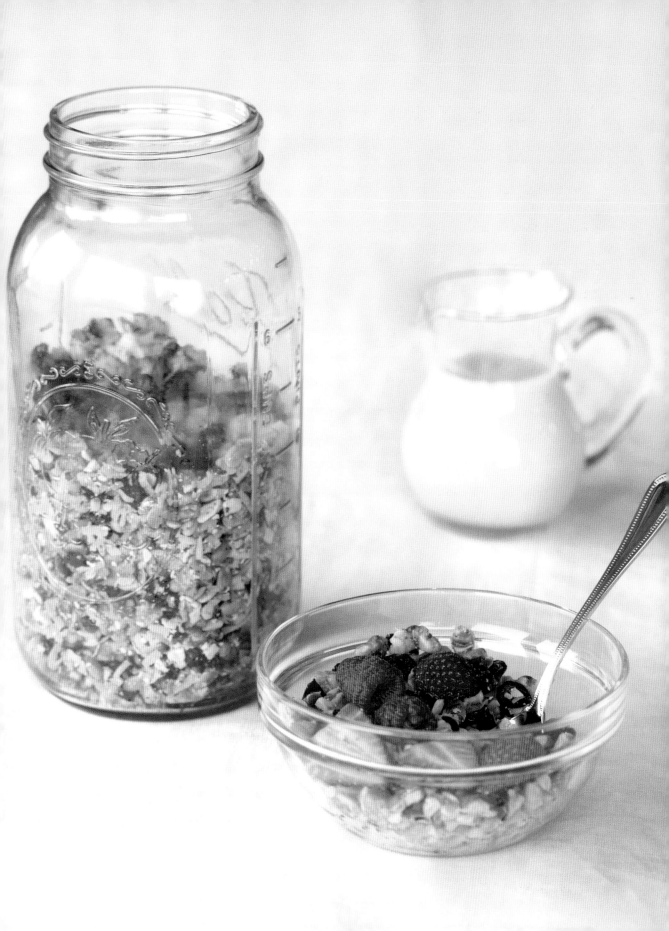

LUNCH & DINNER

FISH TACOS *with guacamole*

*Although the traditional corn-based shells are
missing, these tacos are certainly reminiscent
of fresh fish tacos, with light, bright flavors.*

4 lettuce cups (large whole leaves of
    romaine or iceberg lettuce)
4 fillets firm white fish (e.g., cod or halibut),
    about 20 oz. (600 g)*
1½ cups (135 g) red cabbage,
    thinly sliced or shredded
1 Tbsp. rice vinegar
1 red chili pepper, seeded and chopped
2 Tbsp. fresh mint leaves, chopped
2 Tbsp. fresh cilantro, chopped
2 tomatoes, diced

* *Leftover cooked chicken can also
    be used in this recipe.*

GUACAMOLE

1 large avocado, skin and pit removed
1 small red chili pepper, seeded and chopped
Juice of 1 lime
1 Tbsp. fresh cilantro, chopped
Sea salt and pepper

Carefully wash and dry the lettuce leaves, keeping
them intact, and set aside.

To make the guacamole: Mash the avocado, then
add the red chili pepper, lime juice, and cilantro
and season with salt and pepper to taste. Set aside.

To cook the fish and prepare the filling: Place the
fish fillets in a large steamer basket set over boiling
water. Cover and steam until just cooked through,
about 10–15 minutes (depending on the thickness
of the fillets). Remove and gently flake or slice
into thirds.

While the fish is cooking, toss the cabbage with
the rice vinegar, red chili pepper, and herbs.

To assemble the tacos, add some of the cabbage
mixture to the bottom of the lettuce cups. Top each
taco with pieces of the fish, diced tomatoes, and
a dollop of guacamole. Serve immediately.

STEAMING is a fantastic way to cook fish because it allows the flavors of the
fish to stand out. Really any fish can be steamed; it's an almost foolproof technique
for keeping the flesh moist. Adding herbs or spices to the steamer infuses
those flavors into the fish. If you don't have a steamer, you can poach the fish
or even gently panfry it in a small amount of coconut oil.

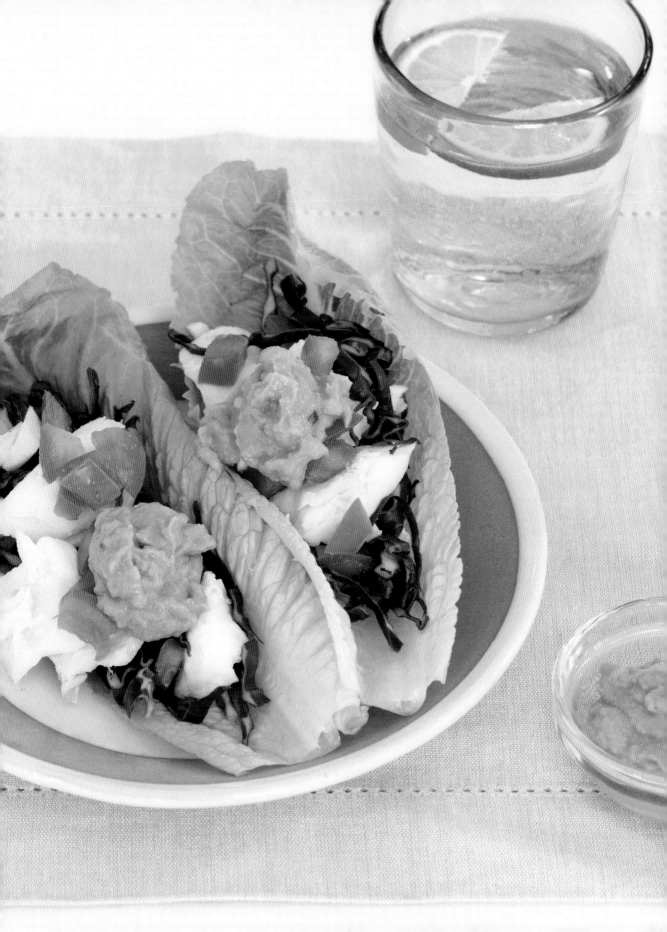

WARM SHRIMP, PEA, SHALLOT & HERB SALAD

SERVES 2

Use the freshest herbs and the best-quality shrimp you can find to make this refreshing salad. The ingredients are the real stars here.

2 tsp. sea salt
8–16 shrimp, about 1 lb. (450 g)
2 Tbsp. olive oil, divided
1 shallot, finely chopped
3 cups (400 g) frozen peas
1 cup (240 ml) water
1 Tbsp. fresh mint, finely chopped
1 Tbsp. fresh parsley, finely chopped
1 Tbsp. fresh basil, finely chopped
1 Tbsp. lemon juice
Sea salt and pepper

Add salt to a large pot of water and bring to a boil. Add the shrimp and cook for 3–4 minutes. When the shrimp are cooked they will float to the surface and change to an opaque pinky orange. Do not overcook, or they will be tough. Remove from the water and place into a bowl of ice water for 1 minute to stop the cooking process. Drain and remove the heads and shells (and devein, if desired) before setting aside.

Heat 1 tablespoon of the olive oil in a large skillet set over low heat. Add the shallot and sauté until just cooked. Add the peas and water and cook until the peas are cooked through and most of the water has evaporated, about 5 minutes.

Add the shrimp and stir to warm through. Add the herbs, lemon juice, and remaining olive oil and season with salt and pepper to taste. Serve immediately.

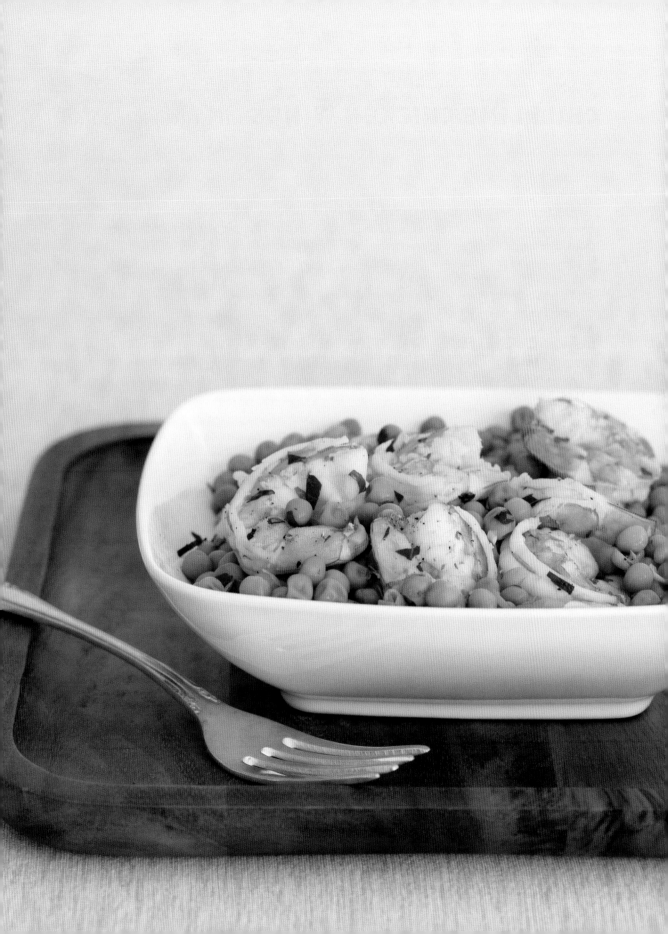

CHILI LIME CHICKEN WINGS *with cucumber salad*

SERVES 4

Some traditions are too good to let go. When it comes time to watch sports with friends, chicken wings seem to be a rule. There's no need to break from your resolve or eat flavorless food—classic foods can be reinvented with a little extra effort. In fact, I think you'll find these chicken wings equally good on other occasions.

8 large chicken wings or 12 smaller ones, about 1 lb. (450 g)
1 tsp. crushed red pepper
Juice of 2 limes
2 garlic cloves, crushed
3 Tbsp. fresh ginger, grated
2 Tbsp. olive oil
Sea salt and pepper
2 Tbsp. fresh cilantro, chopped
1 lime, cut into wedges

CUCUMBER SALAD

2 medium cucumbers
1 Tbsp. fresh mint leaves, finely chopped
1 Tbsp. rice vinegar
Pinch of sea salt
1 Tbsp. toasted sesame seeds

Bring a large pot of water to boil. Add the chicken wings and simmer for 8 minutes. Drain and set aside.

Combine the crushed red pepper, lime juice, garlic, ginger, and olive oil in a large nonreactive bowl and season with salt and pepper to taste. Add the chicken wings and toss to coat well. Cover and let marinate in the refrigerator for 1 hour or longer.

Preheat the oven to 400°F (200°C).

Place the chicken wings on a wire rack inside a large, shallow baking pan. Bake until golden, about 20–30 minutes. Turn and bake another 5–10 minutes. Remove and let cool for 5 minutes. Serve on a large platter with the cilantro as garnish and lime wedges on the side.

To make the cucumber salad: While the chicken is baking, thinly slice the cucumber on the diagonal; use a mandolin or a sharp knife to cut it as thinly as possible. In a medium bowl mix the cucumber with the mint, then toss with the vinegar and salt. Sprinkle with the sesame seeds and serve.

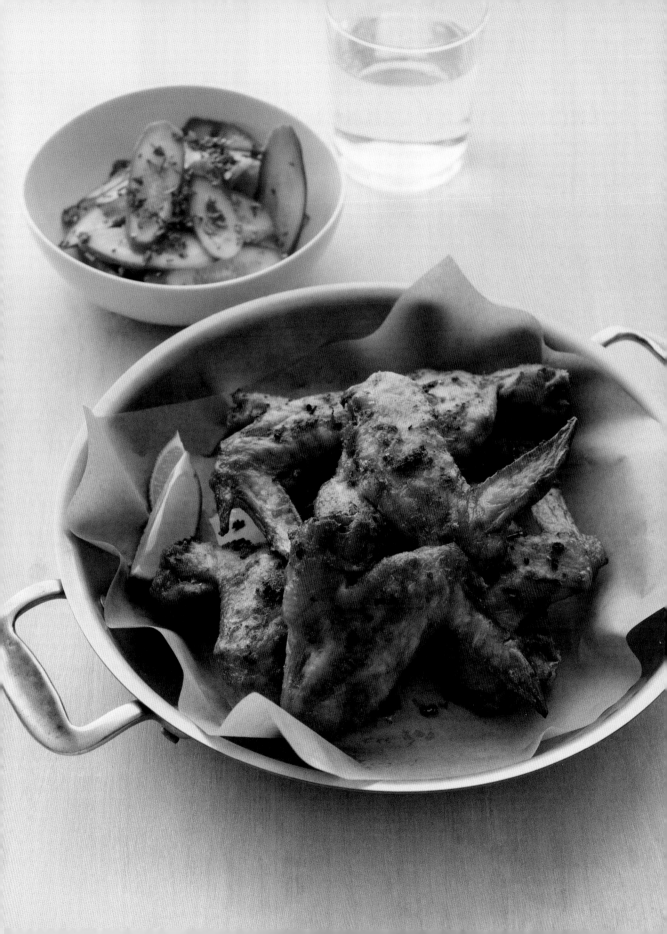

CRISPY, STICKY CHICKEN *with figs & broccoli salad*

SERVES 6

The broccoli salad is made with raw broccoli. Make it before you start the chicken to allow time for the flavors to develop and the greens to soften. For extra texture and flavor, you could also add some flaked almonds or change up the herbs and spices.

1 whole chicken, butterflied, about 3½ lb. (1.5 kg)
Sea salt and pepper
1 Tbsp. olive oil
1 Tbsp. honey at room temperature or heated until runny
4 fresh figs, sliced*
¼ cup (15 g) fresh parsley, roughly chopped
1 Tbsp. toasted sesame seeds

* *If figs aren't in season, use dried figs soaked in a bowl of water for 10 minutes before slicing.*

BROCCOLI SALAD

1 head broccoli
1 clove garlic, crushed
Juice from 1 lemon
⅓ cup (80 ml) olive oil
Sea salt and pepper

Preheat the oven to 375°F (190°C).

To make the broccoli salad: Finely chop the broccoli, including the stem. (You can make fast work of this by pulsing the broccoli in a food processor.) Transfer the broccoli to a large bowl. In a small bowl or cup combine the garlic, lemon juice, and olive oil and season with salt and pepper to taste. Add the dressing to the broccoli and toss well. Refrigerate for at least 1 hour before serving.

To make the chicken: Place the chicken in a large roasting pan on a rack, skin side up. Season well with salt and pepper to taste and drizzle with olive oil. Bake until the chicken is fully cooked, about 50–60 minutes.

Remove the chicken from the oven, and preheat the oven broiler to medium-high. Brush the chicken with the honey, top with the sliced figs, and place under the broiler for 5 minutes or until the skin is golden.

Remove the chicken from the oven and let it rest for 10 minutes before garnishing with the chopped parsley and sesame seeds. Carve and serve with the broccoli salad.

If after testing foods you find you can tolerate cheese, add some feta to the broccoli salad to give it extra dimension.

BUTTERFLIED simply means the chicken has been cut through the backbone and then flattened out. After you cut along the backbone, turn the chicken over and press down on the breastbone until you hear a crack. Alternatively, ask your friendly butcher to butterfly it for you.

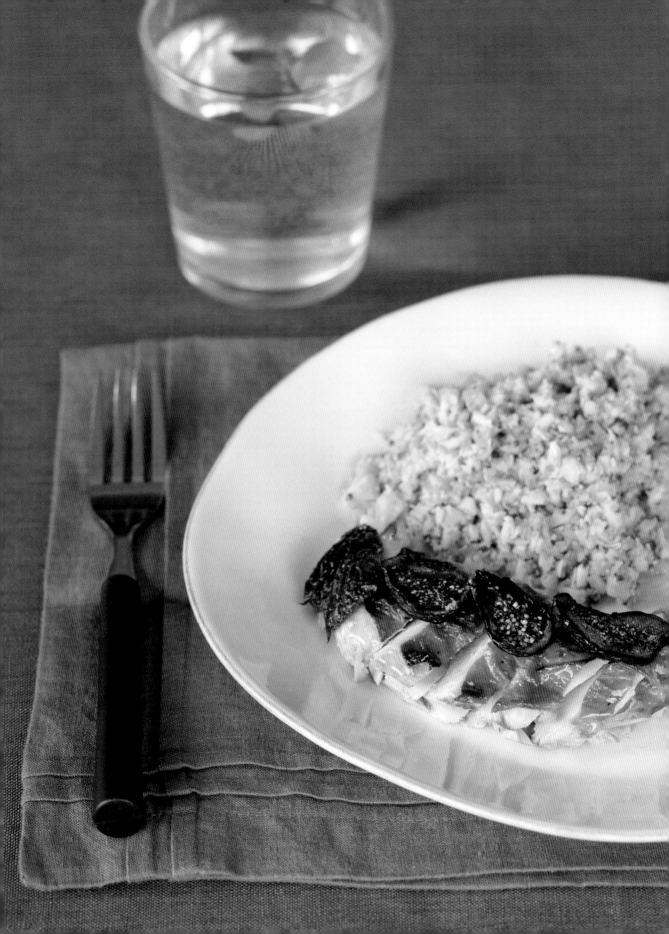

FRIED RICE *with shrimp*

SERVES 4

Leftover rice works best in fried rice; just make sure it's not more than a day old. This is the perfect meal to make after your evening workout for quick carbs and protein to speed refueling and recovery. Use a firm rice like jasmine or basmati rather than short-grain varieties, which are better suited for risottos and creamy dishes.

2 tsp. sea salt
16–32 shrimp, about 2 lb. (1 kg)*
1 Tbsp. coconut oil
2 strips bacon, chopped
2 eggs, lightly beaten
2 shallots, finely chopped
1 small bok choy or 1 cup broccoli florets, roughly chopped
4 cups (740 g) white rice, cooked and cooled
1½ cups (200 g) frozen peas
1 Tbsp. fresh cilantro, chopped

* Shredded cooked chicken also works well in this recipe.

Add salt to a large pot of water and bring to a boil. Add the shrimp and cook for 3–4 minutes. When the shrimp are cooked they will float to the surface and change to an opaque pinky orange. Do not overcook, or they will be tough. Remove from the water and place into a bowl of ice water for 1 minute to stop the cooking process. Drain and remove the heads and shells (and devein, if desired) before setting aside.

Heat the coconut oil in a large wok set over high heat. Add the bacon and stir until cooked, then drain it on paper towels and set aside.

Add the eggs to the hot pan, swirling quickly to thinly coat the bottom of the pan. Let them cook for 30 seconds. Using a spatula, remove the omelet and cut it into strips with a knife before setting aside.

If the pan is dry, add another teaspoon of coconut oil before adding the shallots and cooking until the color brightens, about 1 minute. Add the bok choy or broccoli and cook another minute until just cooked but still al dente. Add the rice, bacon, and peas. Cook, stirring constantly to break up the rice and heat through. Add the omelet strips, cilantro, and shrimp and stir through. Serve immediately.

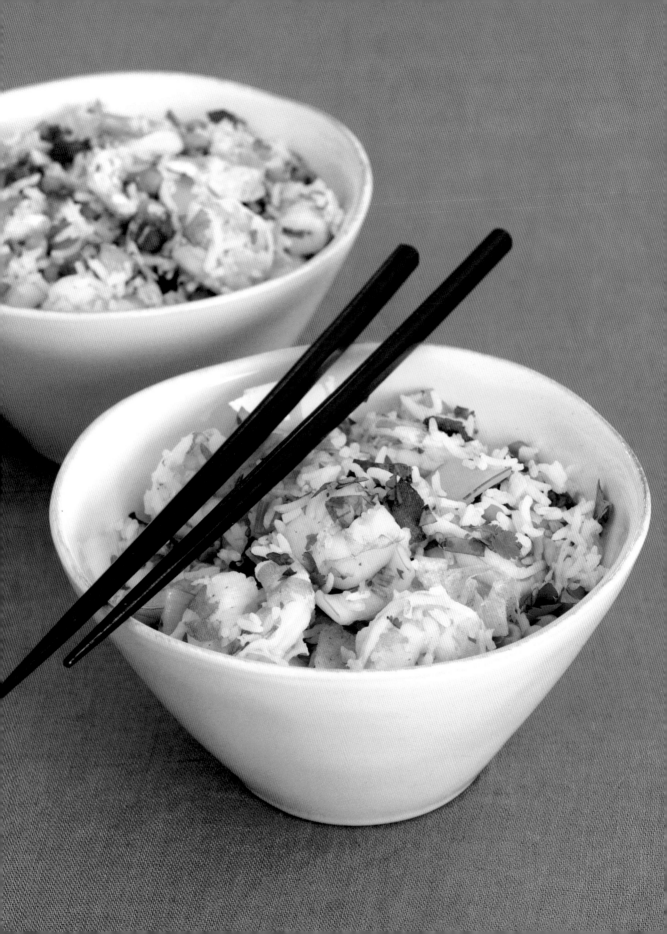

GRILLED LAMB &
POMEGRANATE SALAD

SERVES 4

Sumac is a Middle Eastern spice produced from the ground berries of the rhus tree. It has a distinctive deep purple or maroon color and is prized for its flavor—fruity, slightly tart yet also sweet, reminiscent of a citrus tang. Use this spice in meat rubs and on baked salmon, grilled chicken, vegetables, and pilafs—anywhere you might add a squeeze of lemon. It's a spice that you can be generous with. If you can't find sumac, this recipe is still worth making—the pomegranate seeds and dressing add their own dimension of sweet and tart.

2 lb. (900 g) lamb tenderloin or top round fillets
1 Tbsp. dried sumac (optional)
Sea salt and pepper
1 Tbsp. coconut oil, melted

POMEGRANATE SALAD

4 cups (120 g) baby spinach leaves
1 carrot, peeled and grated
1 large beet, peeled and grated
1 Tbsp. olive oil
2 tsp. balsamic vinegar
Sea salt and pepper
Seeds from 1 pomegranate

Remove the lamb from the fridge 30 minutes before cooking. On a large plate mix the sumac with salt and pepper to taste and roll the lamb in the mixture, pressing gently.

Preheat a barbecue grill to medium-high. Brush the lamb lightly with the coconut oil and cook for 3 minutes before turning and cooking another 2 minutes. Remove from the heat, cover, and let sit for 5 minutes. (This can also be done in a skillet on the stove.)

To make the pomegranate salad: While the lamb is resting, wash the spinach, place it in a large bowl, and add the grated carrot and beet. In a small bowl whisk together the olive oil and balsamic vinegar and season with salt and pepper to taste. Add to the salad and toss to combine.

Slice the lamb on the diagonal and add to the salad. Top with the pomegranate seeds and serve.

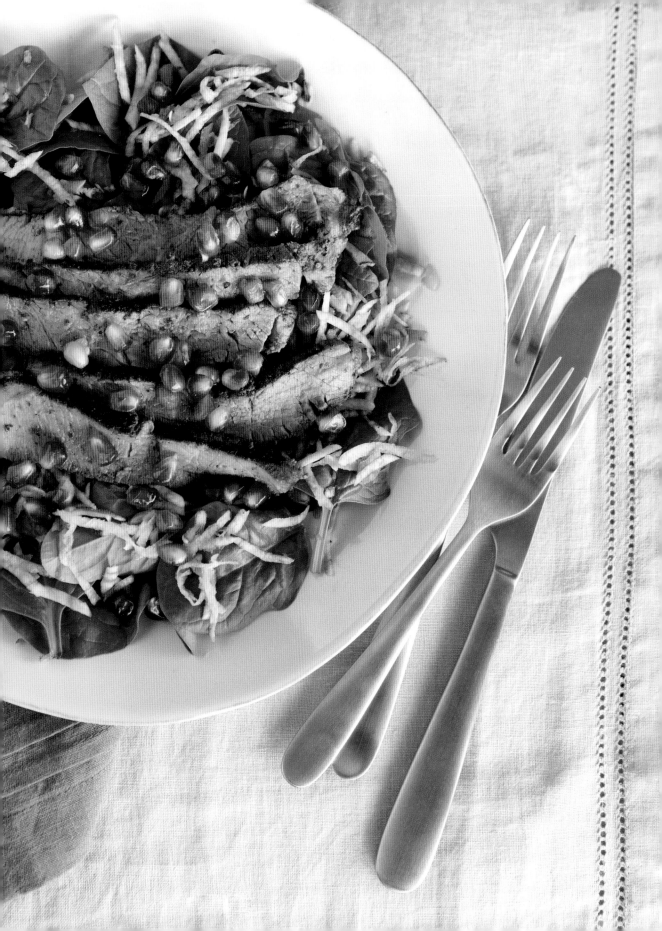

LAYERED CHICKEN SALAD
with roasted kabocha & creamy avocado dressing

SERVES 6

This is the salad I could eat over and over and never tire of it. Substitute other squash or different vegetables as desired. The avocado dressing is also great over steamed broccoli or as a simple sauce for steamed chicken or fish.

1 whole chicken, about 4 lb. (2 kg)
1 yellow onion, quartered
2 bay leaves
Pinch of sea salt
2 lb. (1 kg) kabocha or butternut squash,
    peel left on and cut into 2-inch pieces
    (about 4 cups)
2 red onions, quartered
1 Tbsp. olive oil
Sea salt and pepper
1 cup (40 g) fresh basil leaves, loosely packed
1 head butter lettuce
½ cup (60 g) walnuts, coarsely chopped

AVOCADO DRESSING

1 avocado, skin and pit removed
1 clove garlic, crushed
Juice of 1 lemon
1 Tbsp. olive oil
2 Tbsp. water
Sea salt and pepper

Rinse the chicken, remove the giblets from the cavity, and place it in a large pot with the onion, bay leaves, salt, and enough water to cover. Bring to a boil, reduce heat, and cover. Let simmer for 20 minutes. Turn off the heat and let the pot sit covered for 2 hours. Drain and shred the chicken, discarding the skin, onion, and bay leaves and refrigerating or freezing the bones to make stock for another day (for stock recipe, see page 162). The chicken can be prepared a day ahead and refrigerated.

Preheat the oven to 350°F (180°C).

Place the squash and red onion on a rimmed baking sheet. Drizzle with the olive oil and toss to coat, then season with salt and pepper to taste. Roast until golden and beginning to caramelize, about 50–60 minutes. Set the pan aside. Once the vegetables have cooled a little, add the basil leaves.

To make the avocado dressing: While the vegetables are cooling, combine all the dressing ingredients in a blender or place them in a bowl and use an immersion blender. Add more water to get a thinner consistency, if desired.

Add the dressing to the prepared chicken and toss well.

Wash and dry the lettuce and tear the leaves in half. Place the leaves in a large serving bowl or into individual bowls. Top with the chicken and the roasted squash mixture, then sprinkle with the chopped walnuts. Serve immediately.

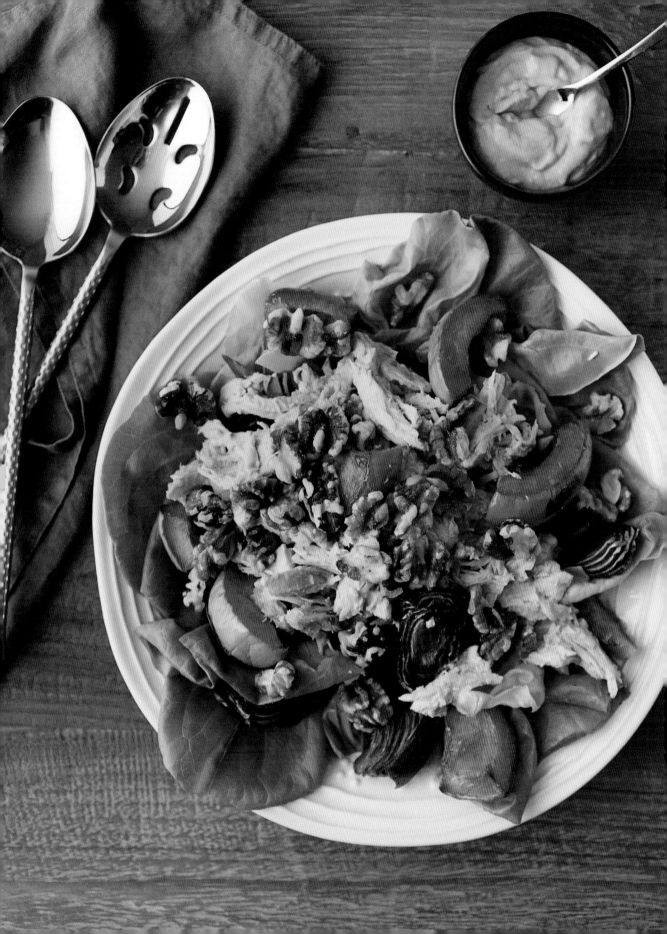

SLOW-ROASTED LAMB SHOULDER
with chard & pan-roasted cauliflower

SERVES 6

Being Australian, I love lamb! I hope you enjoy this dish as much as I do. It's slow to cook, but I make this recipe even when I'm really pressed for time, as it's just a matter of throwing things into the oven and letting them be. Many grocery stores will have bone-in lamb shoulder on hand. If you have time, ask the butcher to remove the backbone, which will make it easier to slice after it's cooked.

3½ lb. (1.5 kg) lamb shoulder, backbone removed
Sea salt and pepper
4 sprigs fresh rosemary

CHARD

2 large bunches chard, stems removed, coarsely chopped
1 Tbsp. olive oil
Sea salt and pepper

PAN-ROASTED CAULIFLOWER

1 Tbsp. coconut oil
1 medium onion, sliced
2 cloves garlic, crushed
2 tsp. turmeric powder
1 head cauliflower, cut into florets

Preheat the oven to 300°F (150°C).

Line a large baking pan with a sheet of foil big enough to cover the lamb too; the excess should hang over the edges. Place the lamb shoulder in center of the foil, season both sides with salt and pepper, and place half the rosemary under the lamb and the other half on top of the meat. Cover the lamb with the overhanging foil and place in the oven. Roast for 6 hours. After removing the pan from the oven, let the lamb rest 10–15 minutes before removing the foil and slicing or dividing into portions.

To make the chard: Steam or blanch the chard until wilted. (You can also cook the chard in the microwave: After removing the center stems, wash the chard. Without shaking off the excess water, transfer the chard to a microwave-safe dish and cook on high for 3–4 minutes.) Stir in the olive oil and season with salt and pepper to taste.

To make the cauliflower: Heat the coconut oil in a large skillet over medium heat. Add the onion, garlic, and turmeric and sauté until the onion is translucent. Add the cauliflower and cook, stirring, until it is just cooked through but still has some crunch.

Serve the lamb on a bed of cauliflower, with the greens off to the side. Serve immediately.

When cooking CAULIFLOWER AND BROCCOLI, always use the stalks.
Some people even prefer them to the florets! The stalks are totally edible any way you cook them: steamed, roasted, stir fried, etc.

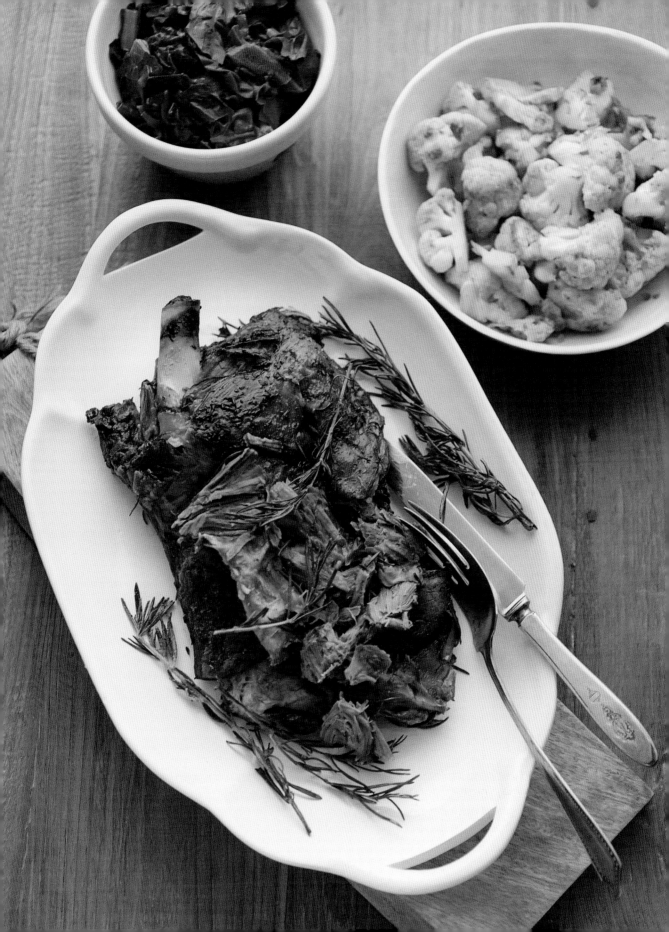

SALMON GRAVLAX *with potato herb salad*

SERVES 10–12

Gravlax is simple and versatile. It's perfect for either impressing guests or as a standby in the fridge: You can add it to salads, omelets, or scrambled eggs. The recipe calls for a whole side of salmon—perfect for a large crowd or for feeding houseguests for a couple of days. For one or two people use a single fillet of salmon—just reduce the ingredients accordingly.

⅓ cup (100 g) salt flakes
⅓ cup (65 g) superfine sugar
⅓ cup (3 g) + 2 Tbsp. fresh dill, finely chopped
1 whole side of fresh salmon, skin on

POTATO HERB SALAD

2 lb. (1 kg) small new potatoes, halved
Small bunch of fresh mint sprigs
6 scallions, chopped
½ cup (120 ml) olive oil
1 Tbsp. lemon juice
1 heaping Tbsp. capers
Sea salt and pepper
1 Tbsp. fresh parsley, chopped
2 Tbsp. fresh mint, chopped
1 Tbsp. fresh basil leaves, chopped

Combine the salt, sugar, and ⅓ cup of dill and mix well. Put a large sheet of plastic wrap on a clean kitchen counter. Pat down the fish with paper towels and place it on the plastic wrap, skin side down. Add the salt mixture, pressing it into the fish. Wrap the fish tightly in several layers of plastic wrap and place in a baking dish. (Juices will be released as the salmon cures, so you'll want to catch them to avoid spoiling everything else in the fridge). Weigh down the fish with something heavy—I put a breadboard on top of the wrapped fish and use anything heavy that I already have in the fridge—and place it in the refrigerator.

The fish will be ready in 24–36 hours, depending on the thickness of the fillet. (The texture will be a little firmer, but the color will not have changed.) Drain the juices and turn the fish over every 8–12 hours, or whenever you remember. Remove the plastic wrap and scrape off the curing mixture. Sprinkle with the remaining fresh dill and slice thinly.

The salmon will keep, wrapped tightly and stored in an airtight container, for a couple of days.

To make the potato salad: Add the potatoes and mint sprigs to a large pot of water and simmer until tender, about 25–30 minutes. Drain and place in a large bowl with the scallions, olive oil, lemon juice, and capers. Season with salt and pepper to taste. Toss gently.

Add the herbs just before serving. (If you add them to the hot potatoes, they will turn brown.) The potato salad can be served warm or cold.

Serve slices of the gravlax with the potato salad and a simple green salad or some steamed green beans.

CURING FISH requires a fair amount of sugar and salt, but they are scraped off before serving. If the thought of raw fish makes you squeamish, keep in mind that salmon gravlax is not raw, because the structure of the protein is changed thanks to the curing mix. Be sure to use very fresh fish.

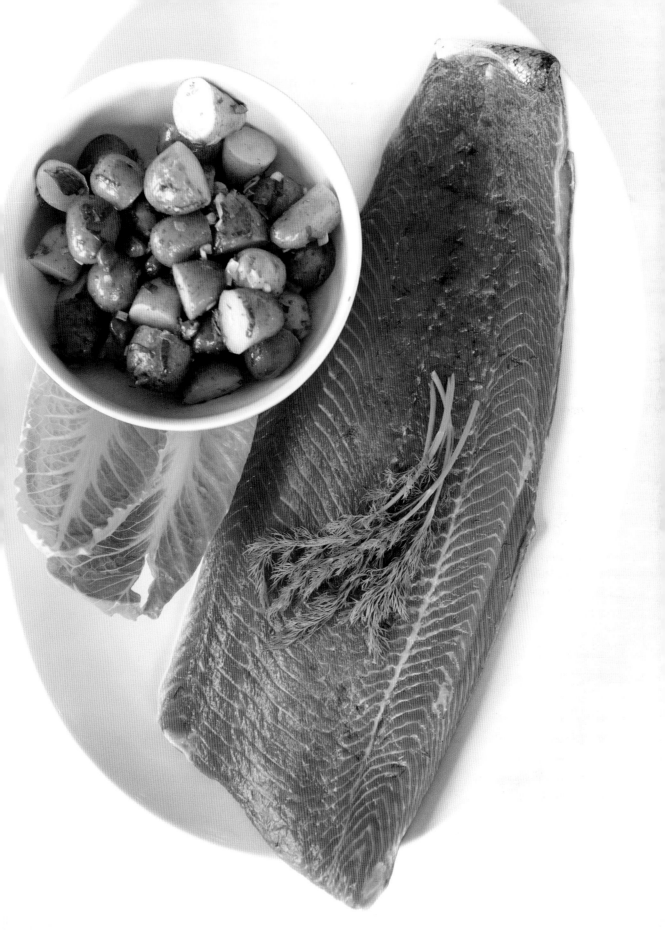

GRILLED FLANK STEAK
with fennel, celery & apple slaw

Flank steak is a cheap cut that lends itself to a good marinade. When meat is cooked with high heat to produce charring, a chemical reaction occurs and heterocyclic amines (HCAs) are produced, some of which are known carcinogens. For this reason I wouldn't recommend grilling every day. Marinating meat before cooking it reduces these toxic compounds, providing a health benefit while also adding flavor. For best results, marinate meats overnight, but if you don't have the time, even an hour or two is worthwhile.

1 cup (240 ml) olive oil
½ cup (120 ml) balsamic vinegar
2 garlic cloves, crushed
2 Tbsp. whole-grain mustard
1 Tbsp. fresh rosemary leaves, chopped
Sea salt and pepper
3 lb. (1.5 kg) flank steak

FENNEL, CELERY & APPLE SLAW

1 medium fennel bulb with fronds
4 stalks celery with leaves attached
1 medium apple
3 Tbsp. olive oil
Juice of ½ lemon
Sea salt and pepper

Combine the olive oil, balsamic vinegar, garlic, mustard, and rosemary in a small bowl. Mix well and season with salt and pepper to taste. Pour the marinade over the steak, either in a shallow ceramic baking dish, a glass bowl, or a plastic ziplock bag. Flip the steak to thoroughly coat it with the marinade, cover (or seal the bag), and place in the fridge overnight. Remove the steak from the fridge 30 minutes before cooking to bring the meat to room temperature.

Preheat the grill to medium. Remove the meat from the marinade, letting the excess drip off. Grill until lightly charred, turning once, and cook to desired doneness. Remove from the heat and let rest on a chopping board for 5 minutes before slicing to serve.

To make the slaw: While the steak is coming to room temperature, remove the fennel fronds and celery leaves, chop them and set them aside, and cut the vegetables and apple in half. Use a mandolin to thinly slice the apple, fennel, and celery stalks. (You can also use a sharp knife or the correct attachment on a food processor.) Place in a large bowl along with the chopped fronds and leaves.

In a small bowl whisk together the olive oil and lemon juice and season with salt and pepper to taste. Just before serving, toss with the slaw mixture to coat.

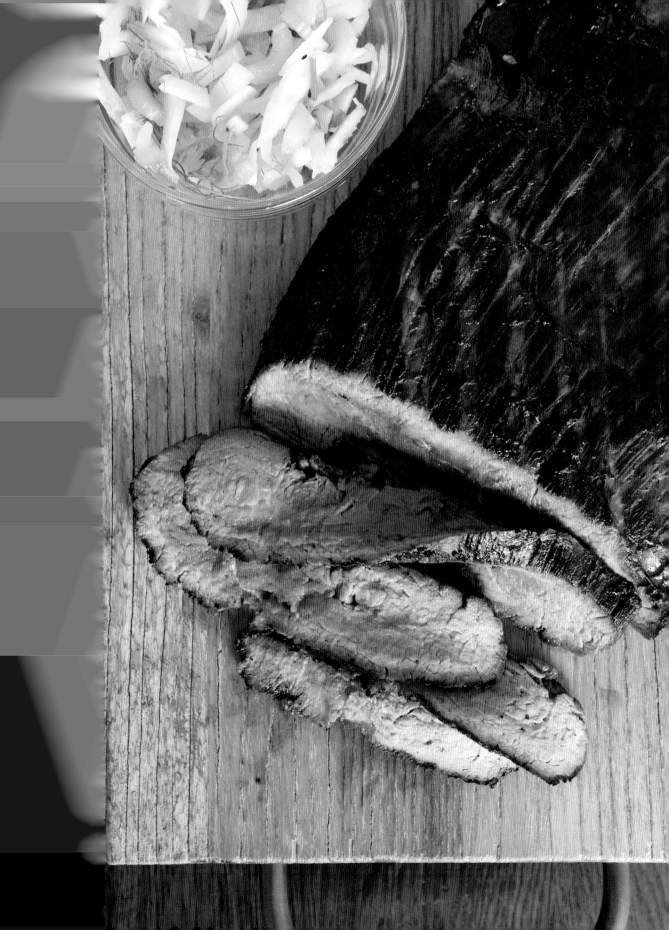

COCONUT BEEF CURRY *with yellow rice*

SERVES 4-6

Curry powder is a blend of different spices, typically chili, paprika, coriander, cumin, and turmeric. You can buy curry blends or make your own. It's a very easy way to spice things up on the dinner front. Curries are always better the next day, as the flavors meld together with time, making them great prep-ahead meals. The turmeric is what makes the rice yellow. Rich in antioxidants, turmeric is a great spice to add to your pantry.

1 Tbsp. coconut oil
1⅓ lb. (600 g) chuck steak (or beef shank), cut into 1-inch cubes
1 large onion, finely chopped
2 cloves garlic, crushed
2 Tbsp. mild curry powder
2 cups (480 ml) chicken or vegetable stock
14 oz. (415 ml) can full-fat coconut milk
1 small head cauliflower, cut into florets
2 cups (225 g) green beans, sliced into thirds
2 Tbsp. fresh cilantro, chopped

YELLOW RICE

2 cups (370 g) basmati rice
5 cups (1.2 L) water
Sea salt and pepper
2 Tbsp. coconut oil
4 tsp. turmeric powder

In a large pot or flameproof casserole dish, heat the coconut oil over medium heat. Add the beef in batches, browning lightly. Remove from the pan and set aside.

Reduce heat to low, add the onion and garlic, and cook, stirring, until the onion softens and becomes translucent. Add the curry powder and stir to coat the onion. Add the meat back to the pot and stir to coat. Add the stock and coconut milk and slowly bring to a simmer. Cover and simmer gently until the meat is tender, about 1½–2 hours.

Add the cauliflower, cover, and cook for 2–3 minutes. Add the green beans and cook another 2–3 minutes or until the vegetables are tender.

To make the rice: In a large saucepan combine the rice, water, salt and pepper to taste, coconut oil, and turmeric and stir well. Bring to a boil, then reduce heat to a low simmer and cover. Cook, covered, without stirring, until the water is absorbed and the rice is tender, about 20 minutes.

Remove from heat and let sit, covered, without stirring, for 10 minutes. Fluff with a fork.

Serve the curry over the rice, topped with the cilantro.

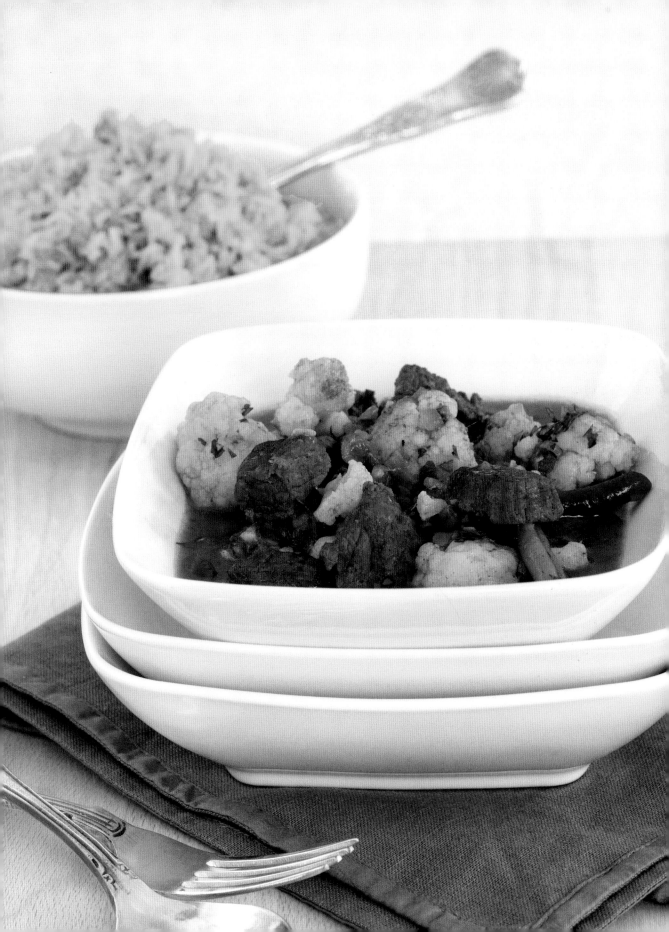

FRESH MUSSELS *in spicy herb broth*

SERVES 4

I think mussels are one of the most underrated and underutilized foods. Rich in vitamins and minerals, they are delicious and incredibly easy and fast to cook. Mussels are also sustainable, making them a good choice on another front. These days we have the luxury of buying mussels that have been cleaned and scrubbed, meaning they are pot-ready. Simply check the use-by date on the package, and don't worry about discarding the ones that don't open when you cook them. That's a myth. Carefully pry them open and eat! Just watch for raw mussels that are already open and toss those out before cooking.

4 lb. (2 kg) fresh mussels
2 garlic cloves, crushed
1 stalk fresh lemongrass, crushed
3 kaffir lime leaves
1 Tbsp. rice wine vinegar
1 cup (240 ml) chicken or vegetable stock
½ cup (10 g) fresh cilantro, chopped
1 red chili pepper, finely sliced
2 Tbsp. fish sauce
1 Tbsp. fresh cilantro, chopped
1 Tbsp. fresh basil leaves, chopped
Lime wedges

Drain the mussels from the brine and scrub to remove the beards if not already cleaned. Set aside.

In a large pot set over medium heat, add the garlic, lemongrass, and kaffir lime leaves. Stir, cooking until fragrant, about 1 minute. Add the vinegar, stock, cilantro, and red chili pepper and bring to a boil. Add the fish sauce to taste.

When the broth comes to a boil, add the mussels and increase the heat to high. Cover and cook for 2–3 minutes. The mussels should open up. If one or two remain closed, that is fine, but if several remain closed, shake the pan, cover, and cook another minute. Avoid overcooking the mussels, as they will become rubbery.

For a light lunch or dinner, serve the mussels in large bowls with the fresh herbs sprinkled over the top and lime wedges on the side. Add rice or homemade sweet potato fries if you need to up your carb intake post-workout.

Other good partners for mussels are tomato-based broths. Cook some onion and bacon in a pan, add some chopped fresh tomato or tomato puree from a can, and throw in some fresh basil and parsley at the end.

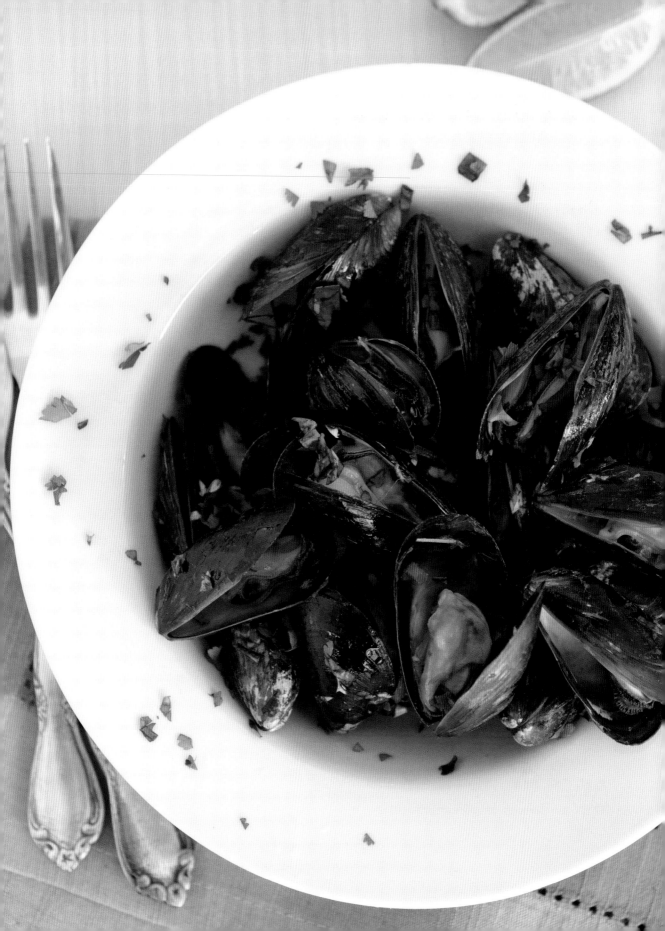

Quick, hearty
VEGETABLE & CHICKEN SOUP

SERVES 4

Soups are so nourishing, especially on cold evenings or after a chilly swim or outdoor workout. Leftover soup keeps well in the fridge for quick reheating, and it freezes well too. You can use lots of different vegetables in soups—select from your favorites and from what the season has to offer.

2 Tbsp. olive oil
3 slices bacon or prosciutto
1 large onion, finely diced
1 clove garlic, crushed
1 carrot, peeled and chopped
2 celery stalks, sliced
4 boneless, skinless chicken thighs,
  about 1 lb. (450 g)
1 small bunch (200 g) kale or cavolo nero,
  roughly chopped
2 medium parsnips, peeled and chopped
4 medium ripe tomatoes, chopped
4 cups (1 L) water or chicken or vegetable stock
3 cups (90 g) baby spinach
1 bunch fresh parsley, chopped
Sea salt and pepper

In a large pot, heat the olive oil over medium heat. Sauté the bacon or prosciutto, onion, garlic, carrot, and celery until softened, about 3 minutes. Add the chicken, kale or cavolo nero, parsnips, and tomatoes, then add the water or stock to just cover. Bring to a boil.

Reduce the heat and simmer gently until thick, about 30 minutes. Use a slotted spoon to remove the chicken thighs and slice thickly. Return the chicken to the soup.

Stir in the baby spinach and parsley and season with salt and pepper to taste before serving.

HOMEMADE STOCK is the secret to making nutritious, flavorful soups. Next time you roast a chicken, keep the bones along with any onion and vegetable offcuts and peelings. You can freeze everything in ziplock bags until you need it. When you're ready to make your stock, place the bones and vegetables in a large pot and cover with water. Gently simmer for several hours—the longer the better. Two hours will make a decent stock, but 24 hours or more will get the most nutrients and flavor out of the bones and vegetable pieces. Store the stock in the freezer or refrigerate and use within 7 days.

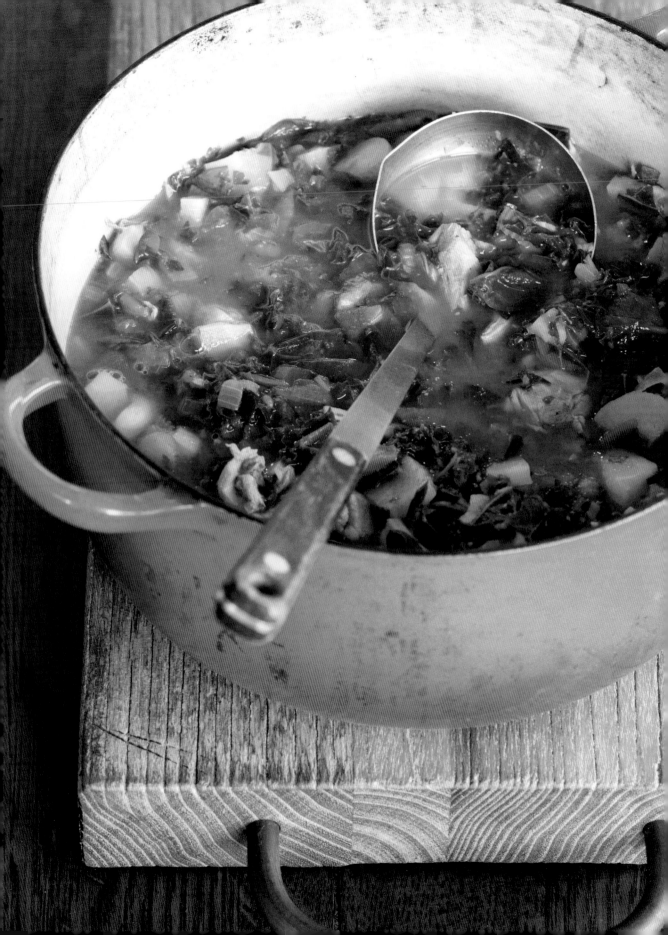

SLOW-BRAISED BEEF RIBS
with cauliflower puree

SERVES 6

When you don't have much time to cook, slow-cooking can be the answer. Light on actual prep time, slow-cooked dishes are full of flavor and forgiving of imprecise cooking, and they take advantage of the cheaper cuts of meat. These dishes also store and freeze really well. Cooking meat on the bone means you not only add lots of extra flavor, but you also get some of the mineral goodness that comes from the bones.

1 Tbsp. olive oil
3½ lb. (1.5 kg) beef ribs (about 6 ribs)
1 medium yellow onion, chopped
4 carrots, peeled and roughly chopped
4 celery stalks, roughly chopped
1 cup (240 ml) red wine
1 cup (240 ml) beef or vegetable stock or water
1 cup (240 ml) tomato puree
2 bay leaves
Sea salt and pepper
2 Tbsp. fresh parsley, chopped
Zest of 1 lemon

CAULIFLOWER PUREE

2 large potatoes, peeled and cubed
1 head cauliflower, roughly chopped
2 Tbsp. olive oil
1 Tbsp. fresh parsley, chopped
Sea salt and pepper

Preheat the oven to 325°F (170°C).

In a large, heavy, oven-safe pot, heat the olive oil over medium heat and add the beef ribs. Cook, turning often, until the ribs are brown all over, then remove them from the pot and set aside. Increase the heat to high and add the onion, carrot, and celery. Cook, stirring, until the onion begins to soften. Add the red wine and scrape down the sides and bottom of the pot. Return the ribs to the pot, turn down the heat to low, and add the stock or water, tomato puree, and bay leaves. Season with salt and pepper to taste.

Put the pot into the oven and cook for 3–4 hours. Alternatively, leave the pot on the stove, bring to a gentle simmer, cover, and let cook gently for 3–4 hours. The meat will fall off the bone when it is cooked.

To make the cauliflower puree: About 30 minutes before the ribs are finished cooking, bring a large pot of water to boil. Add the chopped potato and cook until tender, about 10–15 minutes. Add the cauliflower and cook for another few minutes until both the potato and cauliflower are quite soft. Drain and return to the hot pan. Puree using an immersion blender or a potato masher. Add the olive oil and parsley, and season with salt and pepper to taste.

Divide the puree into bowls, then top with the beef ribs. Sprinkle with the chopped parsley and lemon zest to taste. Serve immediately.

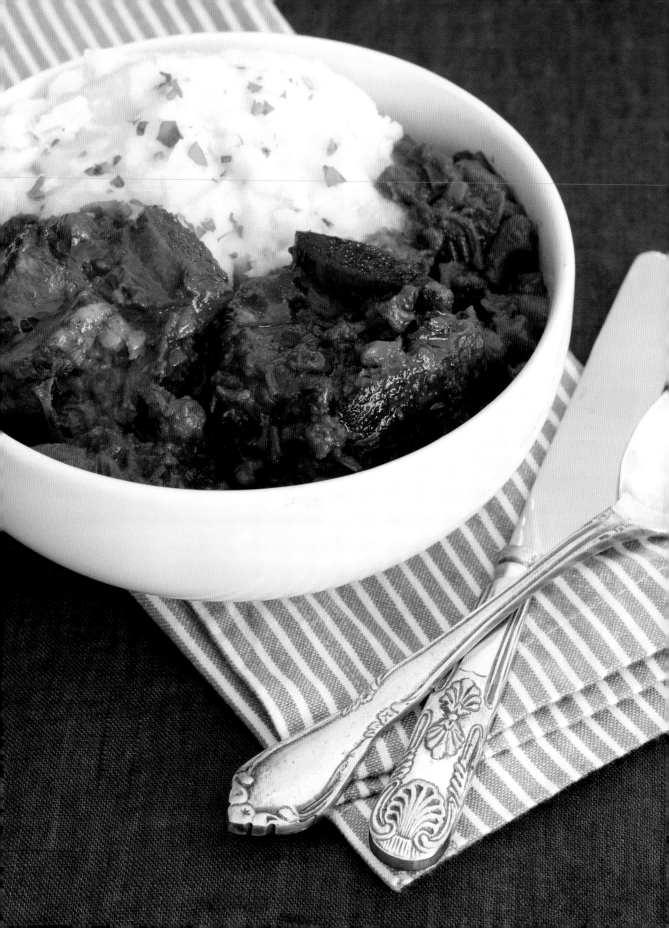

COCONUT CHICKEN STRIPS
with arugula, walnut & pear salad

SERVES 2

Chicken nuggets are somehow associated with comfort food. Maybe it's because they remind us of fried chicken—or maybe it's just the crunch. Either way, this riff on chicken nuggets is a step up from the norm and something you can feel good about eating.

8 oz. (225 g) skinless, boneless chicken
   breasts or thighs, cut into long strips
Juice of 1 lemon
1 cup (240 ml) coconut milk
¼ cup (30 g) coconut flour
1 egg, lightly beaten
¼ cup (25 g) shredded coconut, unsweetened
¾ cup (75 g) almond flour
1 Tbsp. fresh parsley, finely chopped,
   or 2 tsp. dried herbs
Sea salt and pepper
Coconut oil for frying

ARUGULA, WALNUT & PEAR SALAD

4 cups (120 g) arugula or any mixed greens
1 Tbsp. olive oil
1 Tbsp. balsamic vinegar
1 tsp. mustard
1 tsp. honey (optional)
1 small pear
¼ cup (30 g) walnut halves

Place the chicken strips in a bowl with the lemon juice and coconut milk. Cover and refrigerate for several hours or overnight. The lemon juice and coconut milk help soften the chicken and keep it tender while cooking.

Place the coconut flour on a large plate. Have the beaten egg ready nearby in a wide bowl. Combine the shredded coconut, almond flour, and herbs, season with salt and pepper to taste, and place on another large plate.

Remove the chicken strips from the milk mixture, draining off the excess, then dip into the coconut flour. Shake off any excess flour before dipping into the egg and then dredging with the coconut–almond flour mixture. Repeat with all the chicken pieces.

Heat the coconut oil in a large skillet set over medium heat (you want the oil to be about ½ inch deep). Add the chicken pieces and cook for 2–3 minutes on each side or until golden. Drain on paper towels for several minutes.

To make the salad: While the chicken is draining and cooling, wash the arugula or greens.

Combine the olive oil, balsamic vinegar, mustard, and honey (if using) in a small jar and shake well to combine, or mix well in a small bowl or cup. Set aside.

Core and thinly slice the pear (if you do this too early, it will turn brown).

In a large serving bowl combine the salad leaves, sliced pear, and walnuts. Just before serving, add the dressing and toss gently, then serve with the chicken strips.

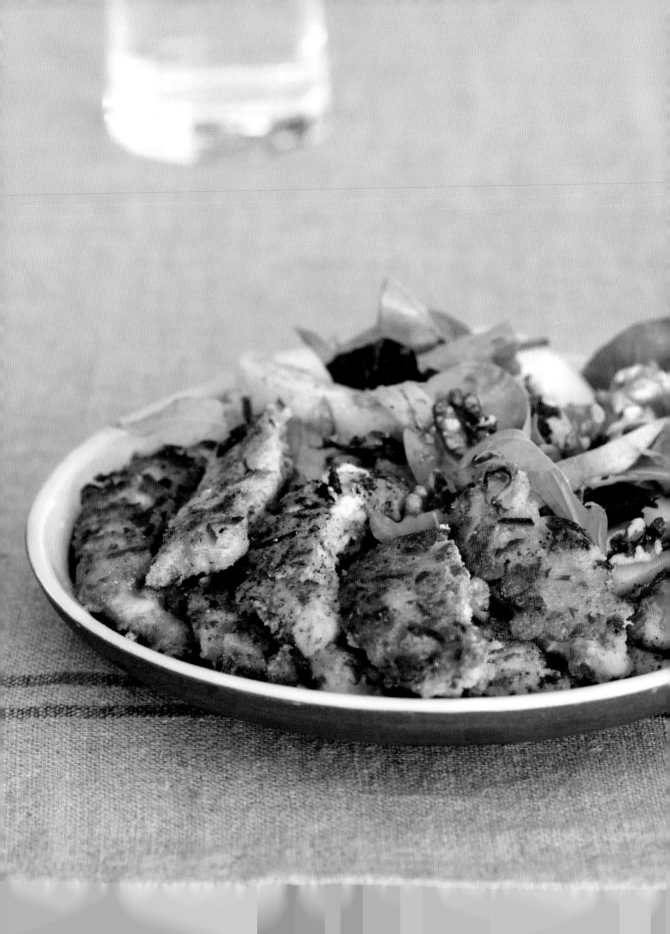

Rice-paper CHICKEN MANGO ROLLS

SERVES 4 AS A LIGHT LUNCH OR 2 FOR DINNER

These rice-paper rolls make a delicious, light summer lunch or dinner. They are quick to make, and the filling can be adjusted according to taste. Try using sliced cooked beef or cooked shrimp instead of the chicken. A green mango will add some authentic sharp tartness, but a sweet, ripe mango also works well and is often easier to find. When mangoes are not in season, you can omit them and use additional cucumber and finely julienned carrots.

4 oz. (115 g) rice vermicelli noodles
1 small bunch fresh mint or Vietnamese mint, chopped
¼ head iceberg lettuce, finely shredded
12 large rice paper sheets
½ lb. (225 g) cooked chicken, shredded
1 cucumber, julienned
1 small mango (green or ripe), peeled and finely sliced

DIPPING SAUCE

Juice of 1 lime
1 Tbsp. rice vinegar
1 Tbsp. tamari sauce
1 Tbsp. fresh ginger, grated

Bring a large pot of water to a boil over high heat. Cook the rice noodles according to the instructions on the package. Drain, then rinse the noodles well with cold water and set them aside to cool.

To make the dipping sauce: Place the ingredients in a small bowl. Mix well and set aside.

To make the rolls: Combine the mint and the lettuce in a medium bowl.

Fill a large bowl with hot water. Submerge one sheet of rice paper in the water for 4–5 seconds, then place the sheet on a clean, wet tea towel.

Top the rice paper with a generous pinch of the rice noodles, then a generous pinch of the lettuce and mint mix, then some chicken and cucumber, and finish with several slices of the mango.

Fold in the left side of the rice paper, then the right, with the edges slightly overlapping. Roll up firmly and neatly.

Repeat with the remaining rice paper sheets and fillings. Serve immediately with the dipping sauce.

Tightly wrap any leftover rolls in plastic wrap and refrigerate. Rolls will keep for 1–2 days.

Makes 12 rolls.

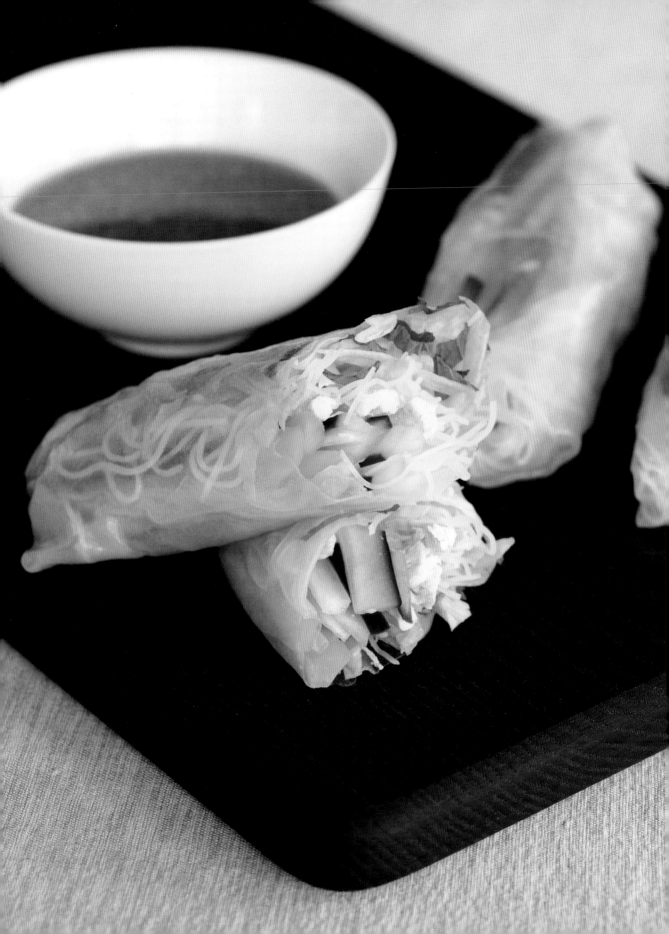

SWEETS & TREATS

These are healthier than your standard desserts, but they are still treats and should be treated as such. If weight loss is a primary concern for you, limit these foods. If you have higher energy needs, remember that more-nutritious foods should be focused on first. Use these recipes for an OCCASIONAL INDULGENCE and as a way of keeping yourself on track.

ORANGE-CHOCOLATE "JAFFA" DESSERT

SERVES 4

Oranges and chocolate are a classic flavor combo. This dessert helps satisfy sweet chocolaty cravings in a quick, light, and healthy way. The mint adds a layer of freshness and accentuates the other flavors.

2 oranges
3 oz. (85 g) dark chocolate (at least 70% cacao)
1 Tbsp. fresh mint leaves, finely chopped

Peel the oranges and then slice them into rounds across the segments. Arrange on a large platter.

Using a vegetable peeler or a zester, shave the chocolate and scatter it over the orange pieces. Top with the shredded mint and serve.

Cocoa beans are one of the richest sources of phytochemicals with powerful antioxidant properties. But it's important to realize that in addition to cocoa, almost all chocolate contains additional ingredients: *lots* of sugar, other oils and fats, and artificial flavors and preservatives. I recommend sticking to DARK CHOCOLATE (70% cacao or higher), checking ingredients, and eating small amounts (two or three squares a day).

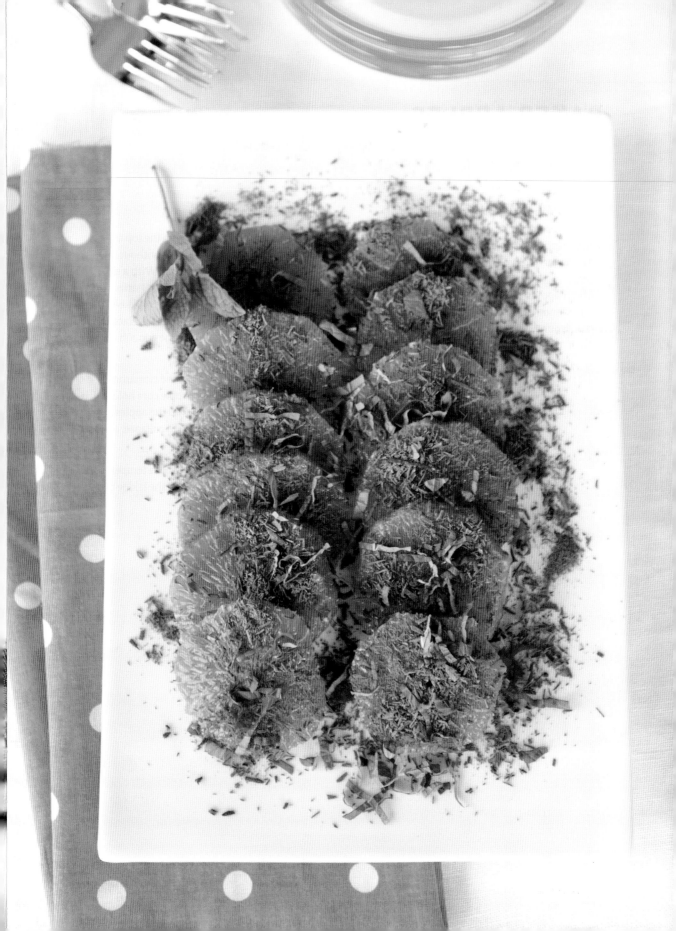

BAKED BANANA SPLITS

Roasting anything brings out the natural sweetness, so these baked bananas satisfy any cravings for sweets. Snuggle up on a cool night after a hard day of training and enjoy the rich, decadent chocolate sauce.

2 small bananas, unpeeled
1.5 oz. (40 g) dark chocolate
  (at least 70% cacao)
1 Tbsp. coconut cream
1 Tbsp. walnuts, chopped

Preheat the oven to 350°F (180°C).

Place the unpeeled bananas on a rimmed baking sheet and bake until the skins are blackened and the bananas are soft, about 15–25 minutes (depending on the ripeness of the banana).

Meanwhile, melt the dark chocolate and coconut cream in a glass bowl set inside a small saucepan of boiling water. Use a whisk to mix well. (Alternatively, melt the chocolate and coconut cream in the microwave using the low power setting and stirring frequently.)

Cut the bananas lengthwise, leaving the lower peel intact, and gently squeeze them open, leaving the skins around the banana. Drizzle with the hot chocolate sauce and top with the chopped walnuts. Serve immediately.

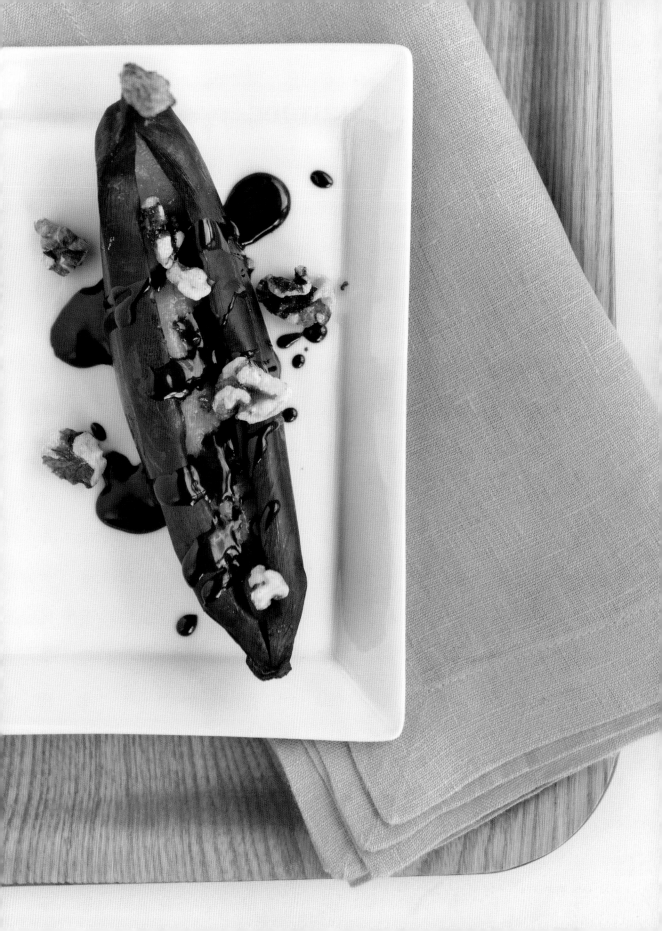

MIXED BERRY COCONUT ICE

This "ice cream" is refreshing and faster than driving to the store for additive- and sugar-packed varieties. Mix it up by using different fruits, and you can also experiment by adding nuts, seeds, or even herbs. Strawberry and basil make a good combo.

1 frozen banana
2 cups (300 g) frozen berries such as
    blueberries, raspberries, or blackberries
¼ cup (60 ml) coconut milk or almond milk

Place all the ingredients into a blender or food processor and blend on high until combined. Serve immediately.

Keep chopped fruit and berries in the freezer for treats like this one and to add to your smoothies and baking.

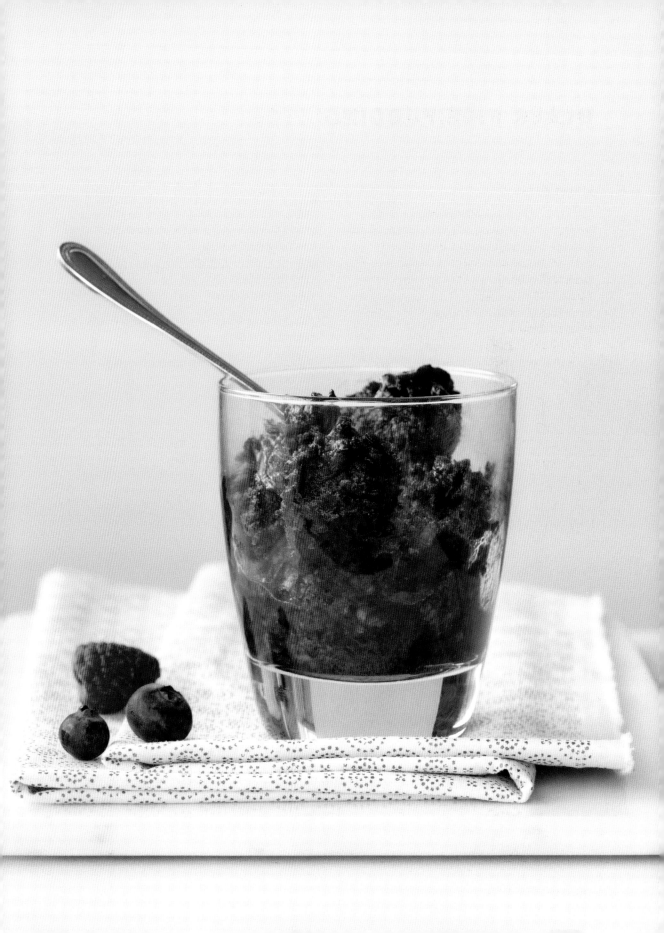

BLACK RICE PUDDING

SERVES 6

Black rice is chock-full of antioxidants, and, coupled with the sweetness of the dried fruit, it makes for a rich, filling pudding.

1 cup (185 g) black rice
3 cups (720 ml) water
1 cup (165 g) raisins or prunes
1 cup (240 ml) coconut cream
½ cup (60 g) pistachios, shelled
1 cup (150 g) strawberries, halved

Rinse the rice well in cold water, then place in a heavy saucepan and cover with the water. Add the raisins or prunes. Bring to a boil and simmer for about 30 minutes, stirring every now and then, until the water is absorbed, the rice is tender, and the fruit has softened.

Spoon into bowls and top with the coconut cream, pistachios, and strawberries.

If you like a creamier texture, soak your rice in water overnight.

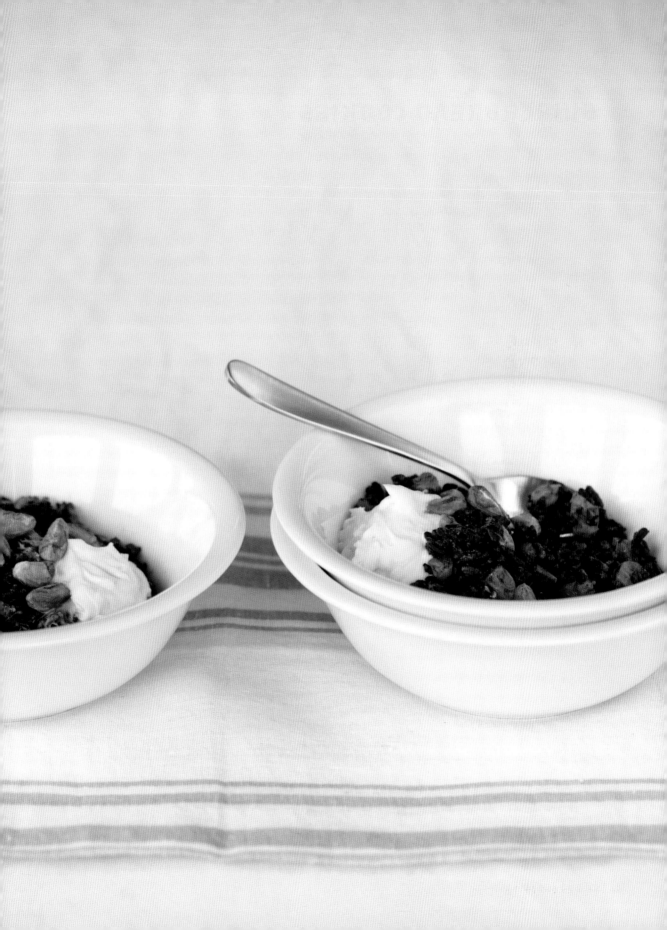

GINGERBREAD COOKIES

SERVES 10

These sweet, spiced cookies are a real treat. Traditionally eaten during the holiday season, I think they're too good to be saved until then. If the weather is hot, store the cookies in an airtight container in the fridge.

2¾ cups (275 g) almond flour
4 fresh, soft pitted dates
1 tsp. cinnamon
¼ tsp. ground nutmeg
2 tsp. ground ginger
½ tsp. gluten-free baking powder
¼ cup (60 ml) coconut oil, melted
3 Tbsp. maple syrup
1 tsp. vanilla extract
1 egg white

Combine the almond flour, dates, spices, and baking powder in a food processor. Process until the mixture is crumbly. Add the oil, maple syrup, vanilla, and egg white. Process again until a soft dough forms.

Move the dough to a work surface and place between two pieces of parchment paper. Flatten with the palm of your hand, then roll out until ⅛-inch (3-mm) thick.

Transfer the dough, still covered in parchment paper, to a baking sheet and refrigerate for 1 hour. If you're in a hurry, place it in the freezer for 20 minutes.

Preheat the oven to 300°F (150°C). Line a baking sheet with parchment paper.

Cut the dough into shapes and place the cookies onto the prepared baking sheet. (If you don't have cookie cutters, the rim of a glass will work just fine.) Gather up the remaining dough and roll it out between parchment paper, place on a baking sheet, and put back into the fridge or freezer before cutting out shapes again.

Bake the cookies until golden, about 15–20 minutes. Remove from the oven and cool before serving or storing.

Makes about 20 cookies.

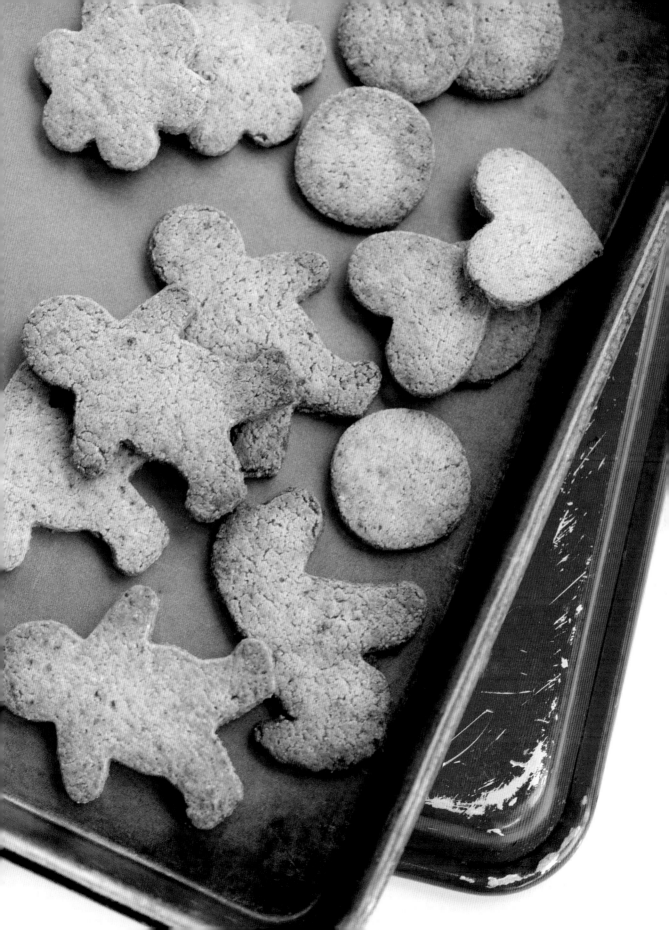

10-minute MINI-CARROT CAKE

SERVES 1

This is a great recipe when you feel like a piece of cake but don't want or need to bake a whole one—after all, it can be a disastrous temptation to have an entire cake sitting around the house. This dessert is ready in minutes thanks to the microwave. I've also used zucchini in this recipe, either in combination with or instead of the carrots.

2 tsp. coconut flour
1 tsp. cinnamon
½ tsp. pumpkin pie spice
1 tsp. raisins
1 small carrot or ½ large carrot, grated (about 3–4 Tbsp.)
1 egg, lightly beaten
1½ tsp. coconut oil, melted
1 tsp. maple syrup

In a small bowl combine the coconut flour and spices. Add the raisins and grated carrot and stir to combine.

In a separate bowl mix the egg with the coconut oil and maple syrup, then add to the carrot and flour mixture. Mix well until just combined.

Spoon the batter into a large coffee mug and microwave on high for 2 minutes. Cooking time may vary with different appliances. If you're unsure, start with 90 seconds, then cook an extra 30 seconds, and then an extra 15–20 seconds, checking the cake with a toothpick after each interval to see if the center is set. Let cool for 5 minutes before serving.

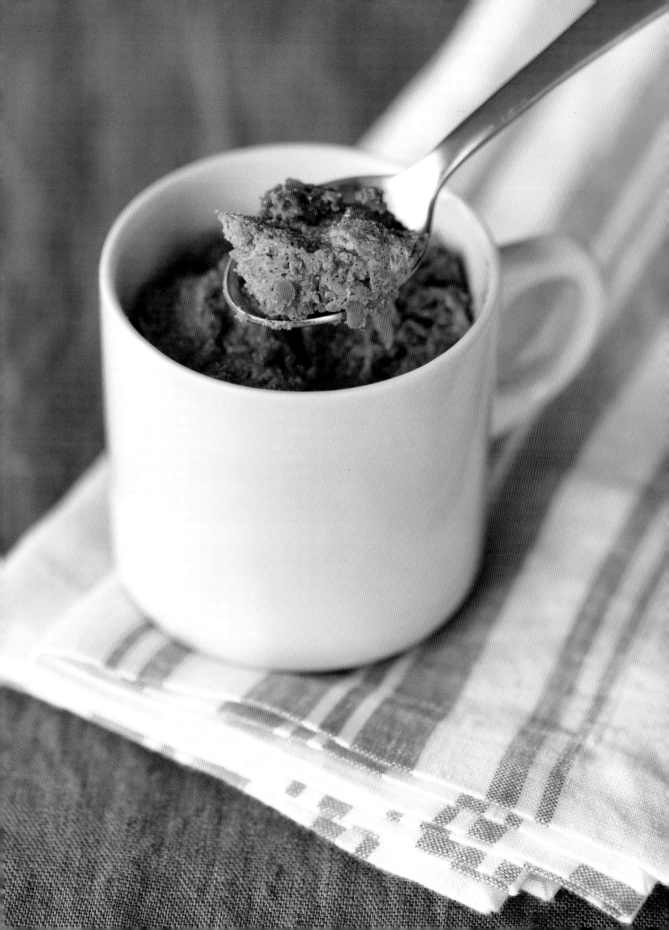

SPORTS FOODS

Sweet potato CHOCOLATE CHIP COOKIES

SERVES 4

Use leftover roasted sweet potatoes in these cookies or simply steam peeled sweet potato chunks in the microwave, then mash well or puree and let cool.

1½ cups (380 g) sweet potato, cooked and mashed
½ cup (55 g) coconut flour
¼ cup (60 ml) coconut oil, melted
1 Tbsp. palm sugar or maple syrup
2 eggs, lightly beaten
½ tsp. ground cloves
½ tsp. ground nutmeg
½ tsp. ground ginger
1 tsp. cinnamon
1 tsp. baking soda
½ tsp. sea salt
½ cup (155 g) dark chocolate chips (at least 70% cacao)

Preheat the oven to 350°F (180°C). Line a baking sheet with parchment paper.

In a large bowl mix all the ingredients except the chocolate chips, stirring until well combined. The dough should be thick but smooth.

Fold in the chocolate chips until evenly distributed. Place spoonfuls of the dough on the prepared cookie sheet, pressing down on the top of each cookie slightly with your thumb or the back of the spoon. Bake until golden, about 20–30 minutes. Let cool on the baking sheet.

Store the cookies in an airtight container in the refrigerator for up to 5 days.

Makes about 12 cookies.

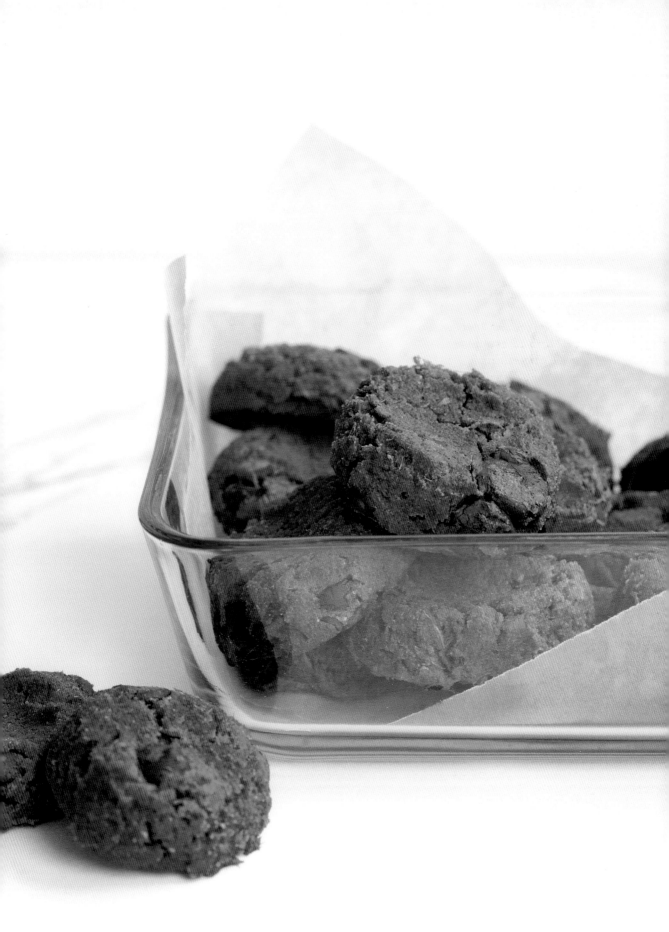

PROTEIN-PACKED CREPES

SERVES 4

Crepes make a great high-energy training snack—simply spread on almond butter and sliced banana or raisins and roll up. Because they taste so good warm, you might also try these crepes straight off the griddle.

4 eggs, lightly beaten
1 cup (240 ml) coconut milk or almond milk
½ cup (60 g) tapioca flour
½ cup (50 g) almond flour
½ tsp. gluten-free baking powder
Pinch of sea salt
1 Tbsp. coconut oil

Combine all the ingredients except for the coconut oil in a large bowl, whisking well to remove any lumps and combine thoroughly.

Heat a small amount of coconut oil in a skillet set over medium heat. Add the batter to the pan ¼ cup at a time, tilting the pan gently to spread the mixture. Cook until the edges start to set, then flip and cook on the other side for another 1–2 minutes. Transfer the finished crepe onto a wire rack to cool while you cook the remainder of the batter. If needed, add a little more oil to the pan each time.

Spread on your favorite fillings, such as almond butter and banana, then roll up and serve or wrap tightly in plastic wrap and refrigerate.

Makes 8 small crepes.

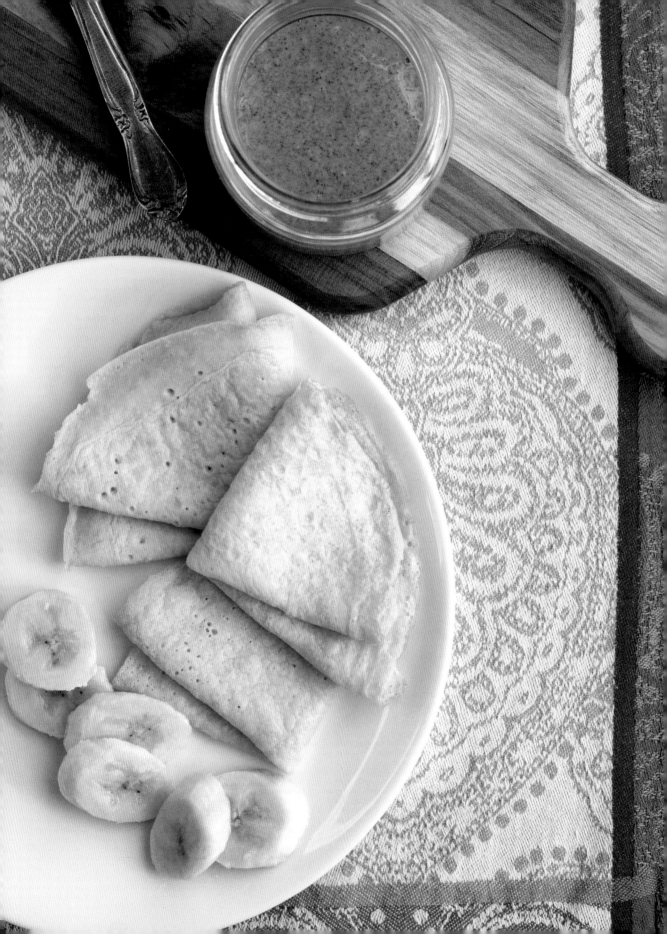

FRUIT & NUT BARS

SERVES 6–8

Change up this recipe to make these bars your own: Use different varieties of dried fruit (apricots, dates, or tart cherries), try hazelnut flour in place of almond flour, add some orange zest or step up the spices, or mix in pure cocoa powder for a rich, chocolate spin.

1⅓ cups (200 g) dried figs

1⅓ cups (200 g) prunes

1⅓ cups (150 g) dried cranberries, unsweetened

1 cup (150 g) shredded coconut, unsweetened

1½ cups (145 g) almond flour

1 tsp. cinnamon

1 tsp. ground ginger

½ tsp. ground nutmeg

2 tsp. allspice

1½ cups (20 g) puffed rice

In a large food processor combine the figs, prunes, cranberries, coconut, almond flour, and spices. Mix on high until the fruit is mashed up and the ingredients are thoroughly combined. Turn the speed to low and mix in the puffed rice—some of it will get chopped up, but the aim is to keep the pieces whole and just distributed throughout the sticky mixture. If your food processor doesn't have a low setting, mix in the puffed rice by hand.

Press the mixture into a parchment-lined pan and store in the fridge to set. Cut into small squares and store in an airtight container in the refrigerator. Alternatively, roll the mixture into small balls before storing in the refrigerator. If desired, roll them in some extra dried coconut to stop them from sticking together.

These bars will keep in the fridge for up to 10 days.

Makes 16 bars or 48 balls.

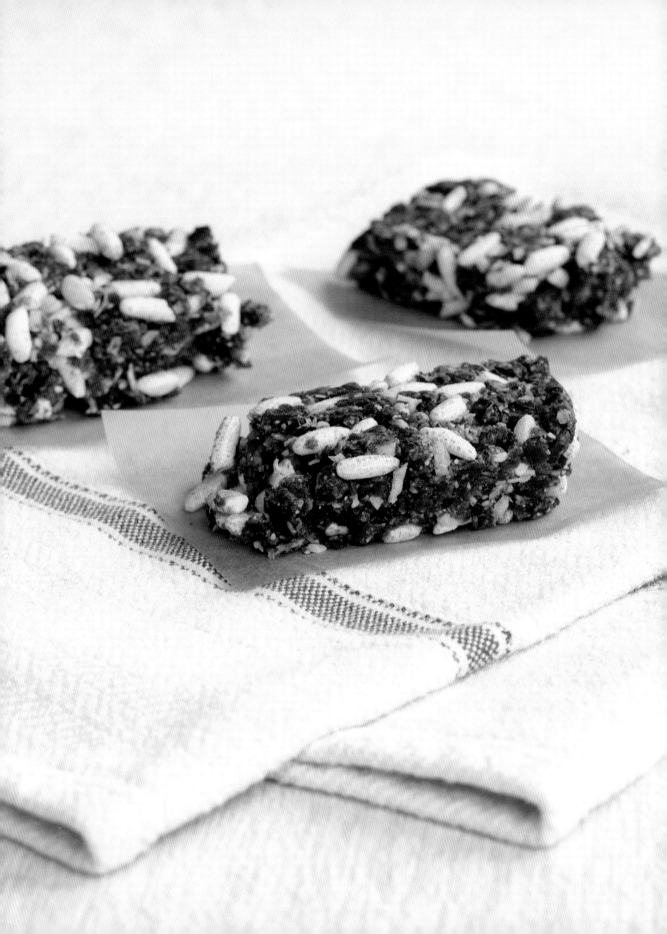

Chocolate cherry coconut RECOVERY BITES

SERVES 8–10

These sweet bites are addictive! I love having them on hand after a hard workout, when recovery is critical and hunger is looming. It's hard to stop at just one, but two or three make a good-sized recovery snack and are just enough to take the edge off and tide me over while I'm preparing a full meal. They also work as a really good after-dinner treat or to satisfy a chocolate craving.

2 cups (350 g) fresh medjool dates, pitted
½ cup (60 g) dried tart cherries
⅔ cup (65 g) shredded coconut, unsweetened
2 Tbsp. (10 g) pure unsweetened cocoa powder
⅔ cup (65 g) almond flour
1 Tbsp. coconut oil, melted

Put all the ingredients into a food processor and blend until well combined and sticky. Shape the mixture into bites by rolling into balls or pressing into a greased ice tray. Store in the fridge in an airtight container for up to 7 days.

Makes 28 small bites.

After completing the base functional diet and testing phase, boost the protein in these bites by adding two scoops of protein powder (e.g., hemp, whey, or rice protein).

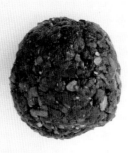

GREEN SMOOTHIE

SERVES 2

I'm not a big fan of drinking your calories, but smoothies do have a place in an athlete's diet as on-the-go breakfasts or snacks. If you are an athlete in hard training and struggling to keep weight on, liquid calories can play an important role. Smoothies can also help athletes who simply cannot get enough energy or nutrients from the solid foods they consume. With all of the fiber from the greens and the skin of the kiwi, this smoothie feeds beneficial gut bacteria.

2 cucumbers, cut into large chunks
2 stalks celery, cut into large chunks
2 stalks kale or 1 small handful baby
  spinach leaves
1 kiwi, quartered (with skin on)
2 cups (480 ml) sparkling water
  (adjust for desired consistency)

Throw the cucumber, celery, greens, and kiwi into a blender and blend on high until smooth. Pour into two glasses. Top one of the glasses with mineral water and serve. The other serving will keep in the refrigerator, covered, for 2–3 days.

After completing the base functional diet and testing phase, boost the protein in these bites by adding two scoops of protein powder (e.g., hemp, whey, or rice protein).

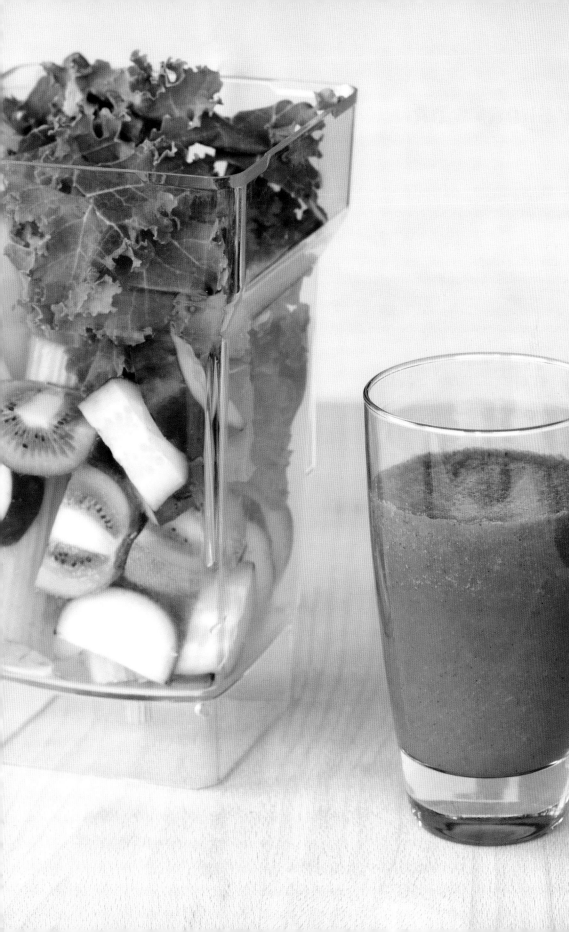

DIY **SPORTS DRINK**

SERVES 2

Here's an alternative to your regular sports drink—a little lighter and a lot more natural. The ratio of sugar and salt is based on the World Health Organization's recommendation for hydration solutions: 3.5 grams of carbohydrate per 100 milliliters, or a 3.5 percent solution. (The combination of sugar and salt is important because the glucose accelerates the body's uptake of the solution, speeding rehydration.)

2 cups (480 ml) water or coconut water
½ tsp. sea salt
4 tsp. honey or white granulated sugar
1 large slice lemon or lime

Mix all the ingredients together well, pour into water bottles, and keep chilled until you are ready to go.

Try other flavors using 1 tablespoon fresh mint, ½ cup fresh berries, half of an orange, etc.

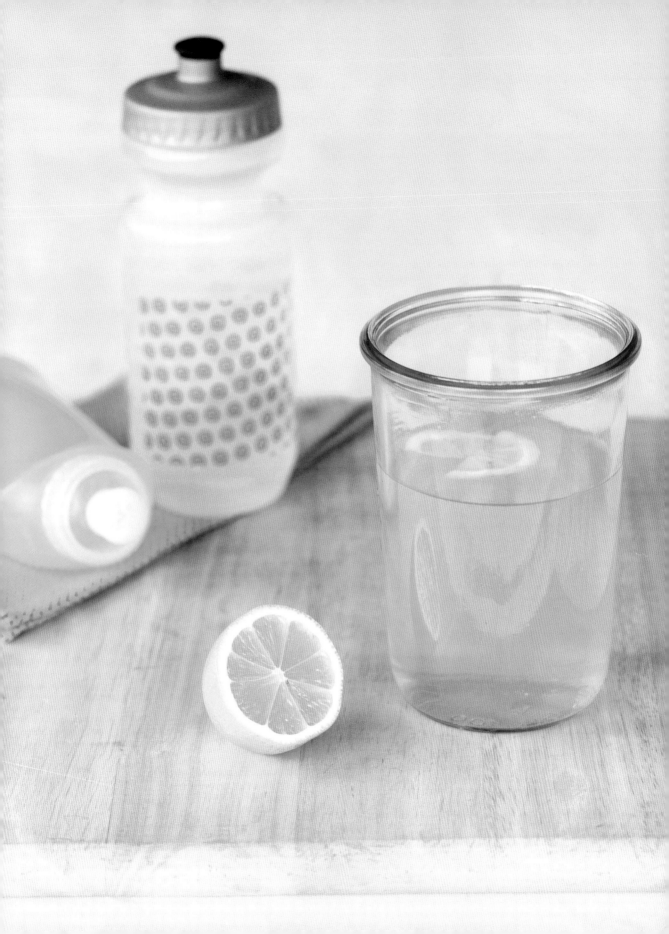

SNACKS

ROSEMARY SALTED NUTS

SERVES 4–8

Roasted nuts make a nice snack, but store-bought nuts are usually doused in vegetable oil and sometimes include preservatives and artificial flavors. It's so easy to make your own roasted nuts—almonds, cashews, walnuts, Brazil nuts, or a mix. And eating them straight from a warm pan is a real pleasure. I have used rosemary here, but you can choose your favorite spices, such as cumin, chili, coriander, or turmeric, to name a few.

1 Tbsp. olive oil
1 lb. (450 g) raw nuts
Generous pinch sea salt
2 Tbsp. fresh rosemary leaves, chopped

Add the olive oil to a large skillet set over medium heat. When the oil is hot and shimmering but not smoking, add the nuts, salt, and rosemary and stir continuously until the nuts are golden, about 8–10 minutes.

Serve warm or let cool and store in an airtight container for up to 3 weeks.

ROASTED EGGPLANT DIP

SERVES 4–8

This dip uses half a head of garlic. When roasted, garlic loses its pungency and takes on a sweet, nutty flavor.

½ garlic bulb, or about 6 cloves, unpeeled
2 medium eggplant, halved lengthwise
1 large red onion, quartered
3 Tbsp. olive oil
3 tsp. lemon juice
Sea salt and pepper
2 Tbsp. fresh parsley, chopped

Preheat the oven to 350°F (180°C).

Wrap the garlic cloves in foil and place in a large roasting pan. Add the eggplant and onion. Drizzle with the olive oil, generously dressing the eggplant. Roast in the oven until the onions are caramelized and the eggplant is very soft, nicely browned, and beginning to collapse, about 45–50 minutes.

Squeeze the garlic cloves out of their skins and blend them in a food processor with the eggplant and onion until smooth. Add the lemon juice and season with salt and pepper to taste. Add additional olive oil for a creamier texture if desired. Stir in the parsley leaves and serve.

ROASTED
EGGPLANT
DIP

CARROT &
CUMIN DIP
(see page 204)

ROSEMARY
SALTED
NUTS

ROASTED
BEET DIP
(see page 204)

CARROT & CUMIN DIP

Photo on page 203

SERVES 4-8

1½ lb. (680 g) carrots, peeled
2 Tbsp. olive oil, plus more for finishing
2 whole garlic cloves, peeled
1–2 tsp. chili powder
1 tsp. cumin powder
1 tsp. ground ginger
3 tsp. lemon juice
Sea salt and pepper
1 Tbsp. cilantro, chopped

Preheat the oven to 400°F (200°C).

Cut the carrots into large chunks and place in a roasting dish. Drizzle with the olive oil, add the garlic, chili powder, cumin, and ginger and toss well to coat. Roast in the oven until tender and aromatic, about 40–50 minutes.

Let cool slightly before blending in a food processor. Add the lemon juice and season with salt and pepper to taste. Add additional olive oil for a creamier texture. Stir in the cilantro and serve.

ROASTED BEET DIP

Photo on page 203

SERVES 4-8

2 large beets, trimmed and cut into quarters
5 Tbsp. olive oil, divided
2 whole garlic cloves, unpeeled
3 tsp. lemon juice
Sea salt and pepper

Preheat the oven to 400°F (200°C).

Place the beets in a roasting pan and drizzle with 1 tablespoon olive oil. Wrap the garlic in foil and add to the pan. Bake until tender when poked with a fork, about 55–65 minutes—the softer the beets are, the sweeter they will be.

Let cool slightly, then squeeze the garlic out of the skins. Place the roasted beets and garlic into a food processor, add the remaining olive oil and the lemon juice, and blend until smooth. Season with salt and pepper to taste and serve.

Serve these dips with VEGETABLE CRUDITÉS (sticks and other dippy bits): carrots and celery, endive leaves, bell pepper strips, broccoli or cauliflower florets, olives, etc. Any vegetable, either raw or lightly cooked, will make this snack complete. All of these dips can be served warm or cold.

RECIPE INDEX

I have not included nutrition information for the recipes because I want eating and fueling to ultimately be intuitive and enjoyable, not a chore. However, athletes do need to get the right balance of carbohydrates, protein, and fat around training, as I outlined in Eating for Performance, page 85. There are times when it's beneficial to eat a snack or meal higher in carbohydrates with the aim of being adequately fueled for a tough workout. At other times it's better to make protein the focus to assist with recovery or maintenance of body weight. And sometimes something light yet nutritionally dense is more appropriate. To simplify things for you, I have grouped the recipes as follows:

Pre-workout fueling. These recipes are higher in carbohydrates and might contain some refined foods and ingredients such as white rice, rice flour, or tapioca flour.

Post-workout recovery. These options pump up the protein to speed recovery. They are also good for athletes with higher protein needs.

Light, nutritious, everyday eating. These recipes are suitable for light training days or rest days when nutrient density is more important than active fueling.

Diet, like life, is not always so clear-cut, so there is bound to be some overlap. For instance, add a little protein to a pre-workout meal or snack and it instantly becomes a great post-workout recovery option. While you develop your ability to intuitively know what your body needs and when and how to best fuel your workouts, you can use these guidelines to promote optimal health and performance.

FOOD DIARY

Keeping a food diary is essential to successfully execute the base functional diet and identify any possible intolerances. Be diligent and honest in your diary and the process of finding your best foods will be much smoother. You can use a notebook or app to record what you eat throughout the day, but whatever system you choose, take the time to create a full picture of what's going on. I like my clients to keep the chronology of the day intact so that the correlation is clear between foods, exercise, symptoms, and other factors. The diary template that follows is similar to the one I use. Here are the important details you'll want to track:

Meals and snacks. This is where honesty factors in. If you eat or drink it, write it down, including the approximate amount. The foods are the focus here, not the nutritional information. Do try to include details of all the foods, including spices and herbs, and whether you cooked at home or ate out.

Training. Note all exercise in your diary, including duration, intensity, and time of day. Consistent records will help you determine when a food is exacerbating or causing an intolerance and when the reaction is simply caused by the exercise itself. It will also help you define appropriate fueling and recovery strategies. Any sports foods and drinks should also be written down.

Symptoms. Pay attention to symptoms throughout the day—e.g., headaches, stomach discomfort, bloating. Rate the severity of the symptom on a scale of 1 to 5, with 1 being barely noticeable and 5 being most severe.

Sleep. This is a vital part of the picture. Food intolerances can impact sleep quality, and poor sleep can in turn affect mood, symptoms, and how we cope with stress. Record both the quantity and quality of your sleep—e.g., "5 hours of restless sleep" or "8 hours, woke up feeling refreshed."

Stress. Rate your stress level at the end of each day, again using the scale of 1 to 5. Stress impacts gut function, immune function, and our ability to tolerate certain foods, and, like sleep, it contributes to the overall picture.

Notes. This is a good place to log your general mood or energy level throughout the day. Are you feeling positive, depressed, or fatigued? Also note anything else you think is worthwhile—the better your records, the sooner you can identify issues and make changes.

THE ATHLETE'S FIX

FOOD DIARY

DATE _____

TIME	WHAT I ATE / WHAT I DID / HOW I FELT	SYMPTOMS RATING

STRESS
RATING

SLEEP (HOURS) _____ (QUALITY) _____

NOTES _____

_____

_____

NOTES

1   G. Vighi, F. Marcucci, L. Sensi, G. di Cara, and F. Frati, "Allergy and the Gastrointestinal System," *Clinical and Experimental Immunology* 153 (2008) : 3–6, doi: 10.1111/j.1365-2249.2008.03713.x; and I. B. Jeffery and P. W. O'Toole, "Diet-Microbiota Interactions and Their Implications for Healthy Living," *Nutrients* 5, no. 1 (2013) : 234–252, accessed August 28, 2014, http://www.ncbi.nlm.nih.gov/pmc/articles/PMC3571646.

2   A. W. Campbell, "Autoimmunity and the Gut," *Autoimmune Diseases* (May 13, 2014) : 152–428, doi: 10.1155/2014/152428; J. Visser, J. Rozing, A. Sapone, K. Lammers, and A. Fasano, "Tight Junctions, Intestinal Permeability, and Autoimmunity: Celiac Disease and Type 1 Diabetes Paradigms," *Annals of the New York Academy of Sciences* 1165 (2009) : 195–205, http://www.ncbi.nlm.nih.gov/pmc/articles/PMC2886850/; and Sapone et al., "Zonulin Upregulation Is Associated with Increased Gut Permeability in Subjects with Type 1 Diabetes and Their Relatives," *Diabetes* 55, no. 5 (May 2006) : 1443–1449, doi:10.2337/db05-1593 1939–327X.

3   A. Festa et al., "The Relation of Body Fat Mass and Distribution to Markers of Chronic Inflammation," *International Journal of Obesity and Related Metabolic Disorders* 25, no. 10 (October 2001) : 1407–1415; and Ichiro Manabe, "Chronic Inflammation Links Cardiovascular, Metabolic and Renal Diseases," *Circulation Journal* 75, no. 12 (2010) : 2739–2748.

4   Jeremy K. Nicholson et al., "Host-Gut Microbiota Metabolic Interactions," *Science* 336, no. 6086 (2012) : 1262–1267; and American Society for Microbiology, "Humans Have Ten Times More Bacteria Than Human Cells: How Do Microbial Communities Affect Human Health?" *ScienceDaily* (June 5, 2008) , accessed August 20, 2014, http://www.sciencedaily.com/releases/2008/06/080603085914.htm.

5   Helena Tlaskalová-Hogenová et al., "The Role of Gut Microbiota (Commensal Bacteria) and the Mucosal Barrier in the Pathogenesis of Inflammatory and Autoimmune Diseases and Cancer: Contribution of Germ-Free and Gnotobiotic Animal Models of Human Diseases," *Cellular & Molecular Immunology* 8, no. 2 (2011) : 110–120; and Ilseung Cho and Martin J. Blaser, "The Human Microbiome: At the Interface of Health and Disease," *Nature Reviews Genetics* 13, no. 4 (2012) : 260–270.

6   Chaysavanh Manichanh et al., "The Gut Microbiota in IBD," *Nature Reviews Gastroenterology and Hepatology* 9, no. 10 (2012) : 599–608.

7   M. K. Ray and S. A. Ray, "Can Modification of the Gut Microbiome with Diet Affect the Onset and Pathogenesis of Diabetes?" *African Journal of Diabetes Medicine* 21, no. 1 (2013) : 7–10; and Giovanni Musso, Roberto Gambino, and Maurizio Cassader, "Interactions

Between Gut Microbiota and Host Metabolism Predisposing to Obesity and Diabetes," *Annual Review of Medicine* 62 (2011) : 361–380.

8   Alice P. Liou and Peter J. Turnbaugh, "Antibiotic Exposure Promotes Fat Gain," *Cell Metabolism* 16, no. 4 (2012) : 408–410.

9   Herbert Tilg and Arthur Kaser, "Gut Microbiome, Obesity, and Metabolic Dysfunction," *The Journal of Clinical Investigation* 121, no. 6 (2011) : 2126–2132.

10   M. M. P. Home, "Fecal Microbiota Transplantation: Where Is It Leading?" *Gastroenterology & Hepatology* 10, no. 5 (2014) : 307–309; and Lauren Gravitz, "Microbiome: The Critters Within," *Nature* 485, no. 7398 (2012) : S12–S13.

11   Hester E. Duivis et al., "Depressive Symptoms, Health Behaviors, and Subsequent Inflammation in Patients with Coronary Heart Disease: Prospective Findings from the Heart and Soul Study," *American Journal of Psychiatry* 168, no. 9 (2011) : 913–920; Nicolas Rodondi et al., "Markers of Atherosclerosis and Inflammation for Prediction of Coronary Heart Disease in Older Adults," *American Journal of Epidemiology* 171, no. 5 (2010) : 540–549; and Yoko Fujita-Yamaguchi, Ren-Jang Lin, and Richard Jove, "US-Japan Conference: Inflammation, Diabetes and Cancer," *Bioscience Trends* 5, no. 6 (2011) : 277–280.

12   Scott H. Sicherer and Hugh A. Sampson, "Food Allergy," *Journal of Allergy and Clinical Immunology* 125, no. 2 (2010) : S116–S125.

13   A. Burks et al., "ICON: Food Allergy," *Journal of Allergy and Clinical Immunology* 129, no. 4 (2012) : 906–920.

14   J. A. Boyce, A. Assa'ad, A. W. Burks et al., "Guidelines for the Diagnosis and Management of Food Allergy in the United States: Report of the NIAID-Sponsored Expert Panel," *Journal of Allergy and Clinical Immunology* 126, suppl. 6 (2010) : S1–S58; and Centers for Disease Control and Prevention, http://www.cdc.gov/healthyyouth/foodallergies/.

15   H. G. Schwelberger, "Histamine Intolerance: A Metabolic Disease?" *Inflammation Research* 59, no. 2 (2010) : 219–221.

16   Peter R. Gibson and Susan J. Shepherd, "Food Choice as a Key Management Strategy for Functional Gastrointestinal Symptoms," *The American Journal of Gastroenterology* 107, no. 5 (2012) : 657–666; and Laura J. Stevens et al., "Dietary Sensitivities and ADHD Symptoms: Thirty-Five Years of Research," *Clinical Pediatrics* 50 (April 2011) : 279–293.

17   Rejane Mattar, Daniel Ferraz de Campos Mazo, and Flair José Carrilho, "Lactose Intolerance: Diagnosis, Genetic, and Clinical Factors," *Clinical and Experimental Gastroenterology* 5 (2012) : 113; Gianfranco Mamone et al., "Proteomic Analysis in Allergy and Intolerance to Wheat Products," *Expert Review of Proteomics* 8, no. 1 (February 2011) : 95–115; and Stephen J. Genuis, "Sensitivity-Related Illness: The Escalating Pandemic of Allergy, Food Intolerance and Chemical Sensitivity," *Science of the Total Environment* 408, no. 24 (2010) : 6047–6061.

18   Fredrik Norström et al., "Delay to Celiac Disease Diagnosis and Its Implications for Health-Related Quality of Life," *BMC Gastroenterology* 11, no. 1 (2011) : 118; and Carina Venter, Kirsi Laitinen, and Berber Vlieg-Boerstra, "Nutritional Aspects in Diagnosis and Management of Food Hypersensitivity: The Dietitian's Role," *Journal of Allergy* (2012) , doi: 10.1155/2012/269376.

19   Umberto Volta et al., "An Italian Prospective Multi-center Survey on Patients Suspected of Having Non-Celiac Gluten Sensitivity," *BMC Medicine* 12, no. 1 (2014) : 85; and Knut E. A. Lundin and Armin Alaedini, "Non-Celiac Gluten Sensitivity," *Gastrointestinal Endoscopy Clinics of North America* 22, no. 4 (2012) : 723–734.

20   Ronna L. Campbell et al., "Evaluation of National Institute of Allergy and Infectious Diseases/Food Allergy and Anaphylaxis Network Criteria for the Diagnosis of Anaphylaxis in Emergency Department Patients," *Journal of Allergy and Clinical Immunology* 129, no. 3 (2012) : 748–752.

21   Jonas F. Ludvigsson et al., "Increasing Incidence of Celiac Disease in a North American Population," *The American Journal of Gastroenterology* 108, no. 5 (2013) : 818–824.

22   Francesco Sofi et al., "Effect of Triticum Turgidum Wheat on Irritable Bowel Syndrome: A Double-Blinded Randomised Dietary Intervention Trial," *British Journal* *of Nutrition* 111, no. 11 (2014) : 1992–1999; and Andrea Carnevali et al., "Role of Kamut® Brand Khorasan Wheat in the Counteraction of Non-Celiac Wheat Sensitivity and Oxidative Damage," *Food Research International* 63 (2014) : 218–226.

23   Allergy UK, http://www.allergyuk.org/allergy -statistics/allergy-statistics.

24   Johan D. Söderholm and Mary H. Perdue, "II. Stress and Intestinal Barrier Function," *American Journal of Physiology, Gastrointestinal and Liver Physiology* 280, no. 1 (2001) : G7–G13; G. P. Lambert, "Stress-Induced Gastrointestinal Barrier Dysfunction and Its Inflammatory Effects," *Journal of Animal Science* 87, no. 14 suppl. (2009) : E101–E108; and G. Lambert, "Intestinal Barrier Dysfunction, Endotoxemia, and Gastrointestinal Symptoms: The 'Canary in the Coal Mine' During Exercise-Heat Stress?" *Medicine and Sports Science* 53 (2008) : 61–73.

25   Michael Gleeson, David C. Nieman, and Bente K. Pedersen, "Exercise, Nutrition and Immune Function," *Journal of Sports Sciences* 22, no. 1 (2004) : 115–125; and Joel B. Mitchell et al., "Effect of Exercise, Heat Stress, and Hydration on Immune Cell Number and Function," *Medicine and Science in Sports and Exercise* 34, no. 12 (2002) : 1941–1950.

26   Lambert, "Intestinal Barrier Dysfunction," 61–73 (see note 24) .

27   Stephen N. Sullivan and Cindy Wong, "Runners' Diarrhea: Different Patterns and Associated Factors," *Journal of Clinical Gastroenterology* 14, no. 2 (1992) : 101–104.

28   E. E. Soffer et al., "Effect of Graded Exercise on Esophageal Motility and Gastroesophageal Reflux in Trained Athletes," *Digestive Diseases and Sciences* 38, no. 2 (1993) : 220–224; and Katrina Parmelee-Peters and James L. Moeller, "Gastroesophageal Reflux in Athletes," *Current Sports Medicine Reports* 3, no. 2 (2004) : 107–111.

29   Julia M. W. Wong et al., "Colonic Health: Fermentation and Short Chain Fatty Acids," *Journal of Clinical Gastroenterology* 40, no. 3 (2006) : 235–243; and Akira Andoh, Tomoyuki Tsujikawa, and Yoshihide Fujiyama, "Role of Dietary Fiber and Short-Chain Fatty

Acids in the Colon," *Current Pharmaceutical Design* 9, no. 4 (2003) : 347–358.

30   Kieran M. Tuohy et al., "Metabolism of Maillard Reaction Products by the Human Gut Microbiota: Implications for Health," *Molecular Nutrition & Food Research* 50, no. 9 (2006) : 847–857; and Robert H. Lustig, Laura A. Schmidt, and Claire D. Brindis, "Public Health: The Toxic Truth About Sugar," *Nature* 482, no. 7383 (2012) : 27–29.

31   A. D. Pearson et al., "Intestinal Permeability in Children with Crohn's Disease and Coeliac Disease," *British Medical Journal (Clinical Research Edition)* 285, no. 6334 (1982) : 20; and Sandro Drago et al., "Gliadin, Zonulin and Gut Permeability: Effects on Celiac and Non-Celiac Intestinal Mucosa and Intestinal Cell Lines," *Scandinavian Journal of Gastroenterology* 41, no. 4 (2006) : 408–419.

32   David Y. Graham et al., "Visible Small-Intestinal Mucosal Injury in Chronic NSAID Users," *Clinical Gastroenterology and Hepatology* 3, no. 1 (2005) : 55–59; and Erick Prado de Oliveira, Roberto Carlos Burini, and Asker Jeukendrup, "Gastrointestinal Complaints During Exercise: Prevalence, Etiology, and Nutritional Recommendations," *Sports Medicine* 44, no. 1 (2014) : 79–85.

33   Herbert Tilg and Arthur Kaser, "Gut Microbiome, Obesity, and Metabolic Dysfunction," *Journal of Clinical Investigation* 121, no. 6 (2011) : 2126–2132; and P. C. Konturek, T. Brzozowski, and S. J. Konturek, "Stress and the Gut: Pathophysiology, Clinical Consequences, Diagnostic Approach and Treatment Options," *Journal of Physiology and Pharmacology* 62, no. 6 (2011) : 591–599.

34   Dominique S. M. ten Haaf et al., "Nutritional Indicators for Gastrointestinal Symptoms in Female Runners: The 'Marikenloop Study,'" *BMJ Open* 4, no. 8 (2014) : e005780; Beate Pfeiffer et al., "Nutritional Intake and Gastrointestinal Problems During Competitive Endurance Events," *Medicine & Science in Sports & Exercise* 44, no. 2 (2012) : 344–351; and Hans Strid et al., "Effect of Heavy Exercise on Gastrointestinal Transit in Endurance Athletes," *Scandinavian Journal of Gastroenterology* 46, no. 6 (2011) : 673–677.

35   A. E. Jeukendrup and J. McLaughlin, "Carbohydrate Ingestion During Exercise: Effects on Performance,

Training Adaptations and Trainability of the Gut," *Nestle Nutrition Institute Workshop*, Series 69 (2011): 1–12.

36 Joe Alcock, Carlo C. Maley, and C. Aktipis, "Is Eating Behavior Manipulated by the Gastrointestinal Microbiota? Evolutionary Pressures and Potential Mechanisms," *BioEssays* 36, no. 10 (2014): 940–949; and N. D. Volkow et al., "Obesity and Addiction: Neurobiological Overlaps," *Obesity Reviews* 14, no. 1 (2013): 2–18.

37 Rainer H. Straub, "Evolutionary Medicine and Chronic Inflammatory State: Known and New Concepts in Pathophysiology," *Journal of Molecular Medicine* 90, no. 5 (2012): 523–534; and Jane G. Muir and Peter R. Gibson, "The Low FODMAP Diet for Treatment of Irritable Bowel Syndrome and Other Gastrointestinal Disorders," *Gastroenterology & Hepatology* 9, no. 7 (2013): 450.

38 Jeri W. Nieves et al., "Nutritional Factors That Influence Change in Bone Density and Stress Fracture Risk Among Young Female Cross-Country Runners," *PM&R* 2, no. 8 (2010): 740–750.

39 C. F. Pyman, "Management of Environmental Diseases: A Current Approach to Inhalant, Food and Chemical Sensitivities, Their Investigation and Management," *Asian Pacific Journal of Allergy and Immunology* 1, no. 1 (2012): 63; and Lena Böhn et al., "Self-Reported Food-Related Gastrointestinal Symptoms in IBS Are Common and Associated with More Severe Symptoms and Reduced Quality of Life," *American Journal of Gastroenterology* 108, no. 5 (2013): 634–641.

40 Joy Anderson, "Food-Chemical Intolerance in the Breastfed Infant," *Breastfeeding Review* 21, no. 1 (2013): 17; Andre Kahn et al., "Milk Intolerance in Children with Persistent Sleeplessness: A Prospective Double-Blind Crossover Evaluation," *Pediatrics* 84, no. 4 (1989): 595–603; and Iris R. Bell et al., "A Polysomnographic Study of Sleep Disturbance in Community Elderly with Self-Reported Environmental Chemical Odor Intolerance," *Biological Psychiatry* 40, no. 2 (1996): 123–133.

41 Katri Peuhkuri, Nora Sihvola, and Riitta Korpela, "Diet Promotes Sleep Duration and Quality," *Nutrition Research* 32, no. 5 (2012): 309–319.

42 Kristine Lillestøl et al., "Anxiety and Depression in Patients with Self-Reported Food Hypersensitivity," *General Hospital Psychiatry* 32, no. 1 (2010): 42–48; and Theodora Psaltopoulou et al., "Mediterranean Diet, Stroke, Cognitive Impairment, and Depression: A Meta-Analysis," *Annals of Neurology* 74, no. 4 (2013): 580–591.

43 Roberta Villas Boas Carvalho et al., "Food Intolerance, Diet Composition, and Eating Patterns in Functional Dyspepsia Patients," *Digestive Diseases and Sciences* 55, no. 1 (2010): 60–65; Roberta Larson Duyff, *American Dietetic Association Complete Food and Nutrition Guide* (Boston: Houghton Mifflin Harcourt, 2011); and Erick Prado de Oliveira, Roberto Carlos Burini, and Asker Jeukendrup, "Gastrointestinal Complaints During Exercise: Prevalence, Etiology, and Nutritional Recommendations," *Sports Medicine* 44, no. 1 (2014): 79–85.

44 Mary Jane De Souza et al., "2014 Female Athlete Triad Coalition Consensus Statement on Treatment and Return to Play of the Female Athlete Triad," *British Journal of Sports Medicine* 48, no. 4 (2014): 289–289; and Michelle T. Barrack et al., "Higher Incidence of Bone Stress Injuries with Increasing Female Athlete Triad–Related Risk Factors: A Prospective Multisite Study of Exercising Girls and Women," *American Journal of Sports Medicine* 42, no. 4 (2014): 949–958.

45 Keisuke Suzuki et al., "The Role of Gut Hormones and the Hypothalamus in Appetite Regulation," *Endocrine Journal* 57, no. 5 (2010): 359–372.

46 G. B. Gasbarrini and F. Mangiola, "Wheat-Related Disorders: A Broad Spectrum of 'Evolving' Diseases," *United European Gastroenterology Journal* 2, no. 4 (2014): 254–262; and Yaakov Bentov, " A 'Western Diet Side Story': The Effects of Transitioning to a Western-Type Diet on Fertility," *Endocrinology* 155, no. 7 (2014): 2341–2342.

47 H. Kolb and T. Mandrup-Poulsen, "The Global Diabetes Epidemic as a Consequence of Lifestyle-Induced Low-Grade Inflammation," *Diabetologia* 53, no. 1 (2010): 10–20; and Begoña Ruiz-Núñez et al., "Lifestyle and Nutritional Imbalances Associated with Western Diseases: Causes and Consequences of Chronic Systemic Low-Grade Inflammation in an Evolutionary Context," *Journal of Nutritional Biochemistry* 24, no. 7 (2013): 1183–1201.

48 Edmond Y. Huang et al., "The Role of Diet in Triggering Human Inflammatory Disorders in the Modern Age," *Microbes and Infection* 15, no. 12 (2013) : 765–774.

49 David A. Jenkins, Cyril W. C. Kendall, Livia S. A. Augustin, Silvia Franceschi, Maryam Hamidi, Augustine Marchie, Alexandra L. Jenkins, and Mette Axelsen, "Glycemic Index: Overview of Implications in Health and Disease," *American Journal of Clinical Nutrition* 76, no. 1 (July 2002) : 266S–273S, accessed August 30, 2014, http://ajcn.nutrition.org/content/76/1/266S.full.pdf +html?cnn=yes; I. Spreadbury, "Comparison with Ancestral Diets Suggests Dense Acellular Carbohydrates Promote an Inflammatory Microbiota, and May Be the Primary Dietary Cause of Leptin Resistance and Obesity," *Diabetes, Metabolic Syndrome and Obesity: Targets and Therapy* 13 (2012) : 175–189, accessed August 28, 2014, http://www.ncbi.nlm.nih .gov/pmc/articles/PMC3402009/; and I. A. Myles, "Fast Food Fever: Reviewing the Impacts of the Western Diet on Immunity," *Nutrition Journal* 13 (June 17, 2014) : 61, accessed August 29, 2014, doi:10.1186/1475-2891-13-61.

50 USDA Economic Research Service, "Food Consumption and Nutrient Intakes," accessed August 30, 2014, http://www.ers.usda.gov/data-products/food -consumption-and-nutrient-intakes.aspx#26667.

51 International Food Information Council Foundation, "2012 Food & Health Survey: Consumer Attitudes Toward Food Safety, Nutrition and Health," accessed August 27, 2014, http://www.foodinsight .org/2012_Food_Health_Survey_Consumer_Attitudes _toward_Food_Safety_Nutrition_and_Health#sthash .jMn4puou.dpuf.

52 USDA, "What We Eat in America," accessed May 16, 2014, http://www.ars.usda.gov/Services/docs .htm?docid=18349.

53 USDA, "Food Intake Tables," accessed August 3, 2014, http://www.ars.usda.gov/SP2UserFiles/Place /12355000/pdf/ficrcd/FICRCD_Intake_Tables_2007 _08.pdf.

54 Michael Pollan, "You Are What You Grow," *New York Times Magazine*, April 22, 2007, accessed August 31, 2014, http://michaelpollan.com/articles-archive/you -are-what-you-grow/.

55 John Casey, "The Hidden Ingredient That Can Sabotage Your Diet," accessed August 30, 2014, http://www.medicinenet.com/script/main/art .asp?articlekey=56589.

56 USDA, "Food Intake Tables," accessed August 3, 2014, http://www.ars.usda.gov/SP2UserFiles /Place/12355000/pdf/ficrcd/FICRCD_Intake _Tables_2007_08.pdf.

57 Robert H. Lustig, Laura A. Schmidt, and Claire D. Brindis, "Public Health: The Toxic Truth About Sugar," *Nature* 482, no. 7383 (2012) : 27–29.

58 Laura A. Schmidt, "New Unsweetened Truths About Sugar," *JAMA Internal Medicine* 174, no. 4 (2014) : 525–526.

59 Margarethe M. Bosma-den Boer, Marie-Louise van Wetten, and Leo Pruimboom, "Chronic Inflammatory Diseases Are Stimulated by Current Lifestyle: How Diet, Stress Levels and Medication Prevent Our Body from Recovering," *Nutrition & Metabolism* 9 (2012) : 32.

60 Susan E. Swithers, "Artificial Sweeteners Produce the Counterintuitive Effect of Inducing Metabolic Derangements," *Trends in Endocrinology & Metabolism* 24, no. 9 (2013) : 431–441.

61 Tanya L. Blasbalg et al., "Changes in Consumption of Omega-3 and Omega-6 Fatty Acids in the United States During the 20th Century," *American Journal of Clinical Nutrition* 93, no. 5 (2011) : 950–962; E. Patterson et al., "Health Implications of High Dietary Omega-6 Polyunsaturated Fatty Acids," *Journal of Nutrition and Metabolism* 5 (2012) : 1–16; doi: 10.1155/2012/539426; and Artemis P. Simopoulos, "Evolutionary Aspects of Diet: The Omega-6/Omega-3 Ratio and the Brain." *Molecular Neurobiology* 44, no. 2 (2011) : 203–215.

62 Cynthia A. Daley et al., "A Review of Fatty Acid Profiles and Antioxidant Content in Grass-Fed and Grain-Fed Beef," *Nutrition Journal* 9, no. 1 (2010) : 10.

63 Amit Kunwar and K. I. Priyadarsini, "Free Radicals, Oxidative Stress and Importance of Antioxidants in Human Health," *Journal of Medical and Allied Sciences* 1, no. 2 (2011) : 53–60; and Charlotte Mithril et al., "Guidelines for the New Nordic Diet," *Public Health Nutrition* 15, no. 10 (2012) : 1941–1947.

64 Emilio Ros, Linda C. Tapsell, and Joan Sabaté, "Nuts and Berries for Heart Health," *Current Atherosclerosis Reports* 12, no. 6 (2010) : 397–406; and Joe A. Vinson and Yuxing Cai, "Nuts, Especially Walnuts, Have Both Antioxidant Quantity and Efficacy and Exhibit Significant Potential Health Benefits," *Food & Function* 3, no. 2 (2012) : 134–140.

65 Vellingiri Vadivel, Catherine N. Kunyanga, and Hans K. Biesalski, "Health Benefits of Nut Consumption with Special Reference to Body Weight Control," *Nutrition* 28, no. 11 (2012) : 1089–1097.

66 Patty W. Siri-Tarino et al., "Meta-Analysis of Prospective Cohort Studies Evaluating the Association of Saturated Fat with Cardiovascular Disease," *American Journal of Clinical Nutrition* 91, no. 3 (March 2010) : 535–546.

67 Ibid.

68 Donald Craig Willcox, Giovanni Scapagnini, and Bradley J. Willcox, "Healthy Aging Diets Other Than the Mediterranean: A Focus on the Okinawan Diet," *Mechanisms of Ageing and Development* 136 (2014) : 148–162; and Alan C. Logan, Martin A. Katzman, and Vicent Balanzá-Martínez, "Natural Environments, Ancestral Diets, and Microbial Ecology: Is There a Modern 'Paleo-Deficit Disorder'? Part I," *Journal of Physiological Anthropology* 34, no. 1 (2015) : 1.

69 Alberto Rubio-Tapia et al., "The Prevalence of Celiac Disease in the United States," *American Journal of Gastroenterology* 107, no. 10 (2012) : 1538–1544; and Fredrik Norström et al., "Delay to Celiac Disease Diagnosis and Its Implications for Health-Related Quality of Life," *BMC Gastroenterology* 11, no. 1 (2011) : 118.

70 Christina L. Ohland and Wallace K. MacNaughton, "Probiotic Bacteria and Intestinal Epithelial Barrier Function," *American Journal of Physiology: Gastrointestinal and Liver Physiology* 298, no. 6 (2010) : G807–G819.

71 Alessio Fasano, "Leaky Gut and Autoimmune Diseases," *Clinical Reviews in Allergy & Immunology* 42, no. 1 (2012) : 71–78; and David M. Brady, "Molecular Mimicry, the Hygiene Hypothesis, Stealth Infections and Other Examples of Disconnect Between Medical Research and the Practice of Clinical Medicine in Autoimmune Disease," *Open Journal of Rheumatology and Autoimmune Diseases* 3 (2013) : 33.

72 Juan P. Ortiz-Sánchez, Francisco Cabrera-Chávez, and Ana M. Calderón de la Barca, "Maize Prolamins Could Induce a Gluten-Like Cellular Immune Response in Some Celiac Disease Patients," *Nutrients* 5, no. 10 (2013) : 4174–4183; and Sinéad Golley et al., "Motivations for Avoiding Wheat Consumption in Australia: Results from a Population Survey," *Public Health Nutrition* 18, no. 3 (2015) : 490–499.

73 Jessica R. Biesiekierski et al., "No Effects of Gluten in Patients with Self-Reported Non-Celiac Gluten Sensitivity After Dietary Reduction of Fermentable, Poorly Absorbed, Short-Chain Carbohydrates," *Gastroenterology* 145, no. 2 (2013) : 320–328; and B. Zanini et al., "PTH-111 'Non Celiac Gluten Sensitivity' (NCGS) Is Uncommon in Patients Spontaneously Adhering to Gluten Free Diet (GFD) , and Is Outnumbered by 'FODMAPs Sensitivity,'" *Gut* 63, suppl. 1 (2014) : A260.

74 Helena Malmström et al., "High Frequency of Lactose Intolerance in a Prehistoric Hunter-Gatherer Population in Northern Europe," *BMC Evolutionary Biology* 10, no. 1 (2010) : 89; and Pascale Gerbault et al., "Evolution of Lactase Persistence: An Example of Human Niche Construction," *Philosophical Transactions of the Royal Society B: Biological Sciences* 366, no. 1566 (2011) : 863–877.

75 Theodore M. Bayless and Norton S. Rosensweig, "A Racial Difference in Incidence of Lactase Deficiency: A Survey of Milk Intolerance and Lactase Deficiency in Healthy Adult Males," *JAMA* 197, no. 12 (1966) : 968–972.

76 Aasma Shaukat et al., "Systematic Review: Effective Management Strategies for Lactose Intolerance," *Annals of Internal Medicine* 152, no. 12 (2010) : 797–803; and Robert P. Heaney, "Dairy Intake, Dietary Adequacy, and Lactose Intolerance," *Advances in Nutrition: An International Review Journal* 4, no. 2 (2013) : 151–156.

77 Shaukat et al., "Systematic Review," 797–803 (see note 76) ; and Robert P. Heaney, "Dairy Intake, Dietary Adequacy, and Lactose Intolerance," *Advances in Nutrition* 4, no. 2 (2013) : 151–156.

78 Sarath Gopalan, "Cow's Milk Protein Allergy and Intolerance," *Treatment & Prognosis in Pediatrics* (2013) :

181; and Celso Eduardo Olivier et al., "Is It Just Lactose Intolerance?" *Allergy and Asthma Proceedings* 33, no. 5 (2012) : 432–436.

79   Ibid.

80   Riku Nikander et al., "Targeted Exercise Against Osteoporosis: A Systematic Review and Meta-Analysis for Optimising Bone Strength Throughout Life," *BMC Medicine* 8, no. 1 (2010) : 47; and Paul Lips and Natasja M. van Schoor, "The Effect of Vitamin D on Bone and Osteoporosis," *Best Practice & Research Clinical Endocrinology & Metabolism* 25, no. 4 (2011) : 585–591.

81   Ruth Harvie, "A Reduction in FODMAP Intake Correlates Strongly with a Reduction in IBS Symptoms: The FIBS Study," dissertation, University of Otago, 2014; and R. H. De Roest et al., "The Low FODMAP Diet Improves Gastrointestinal Symptoms in Patients with Irritable Bowel Syndrome: A Prospective Study," *International Journal of Clinical Practice* 67, no. 9 (2013) : 895–903.

82   Low FODMAP Diet for Irritable Bowel Syndrome, http://www.med.monash.edu.au/cecs/gastro/fodmap/.

83   Chloé Melchior et al., "Symptomatic Fructose Malabsorption in Irritable Bowel Syndrome: A Prospective Study," *United European Gastroenterology Journal* 2, no. 2 (April 2014) : 131–137; doi: 10.1177/2050640614521124; Jacqueline S. Barrett, "Extending Our Knowledge of Fermentable, Short-Chain Carbohydrates for Managing Gastrointestinal Symptoms," *Nutrition in Clinical Practice* 28, no. 3 (2013) : 300–306; Justin D. Roberts et al., "Assessing a Commercially Available Sports Drink on Exogenous Carbohydrate Oxidation, Fluid Delivery and Sustained Exercise Performance," *Journal of the International Society of Sports Nutrition* 11, no. 1 (2014) : 1–14; and Asker E. Jeukendrup, "Nutrition for Endurance Sports: Marathon, Triathlon, and Road Cycling," *Journal of Sports Sciences* 29, suppl. 1 (2011) : S91–S99.

84   Felicity Lawrence, "Should We Worry About Soya in Our Food?" *The Guardian*, July 25, 2006, accessed August 24, 2014, http://www.theguardian.com/news/2006/jul/25/food.foodanddrink.

85   Patricia Salen and Michel De Lorgeril, "The Okinawan Diet: A Modern View of an Ancestral Healthy Lifestyle," *Healthy Agriculture, Healthy Nutrition, Healthy People* 102 (2011) : 114–123; and J. A. Fleming, S. Holligan, and P. M. Kris-Etherton, "Dietary Patterns That Decrease Cardiovascular Disease and Increase Longevity," *Journal of Clinical & Experimental Cardiology* 6 (2013) : 2.

86   C. Xiao, "Health Effects of Soy Protein and Iso-flavones in Humans." *Journal of Nutrition* 138, no. 6 (2008) : 1244S–1249S; and C. D'Adamo and A. Sahin, "Soy Foods and Supplementation: A Review of Commonly Perceived Health Benefits and Risks," *Alternative Therapies in Health and Medicine* 20 (2014) : 39–51.

87   S. Malakar and S. Bhattacharya, "Minding the Greens: Role of Dietary Salicylates in Common Behavioural Health Conditions," *Acta Alimentaria* 43, no. 2 (2014) : 344–356; and S. Dengate, "Food Intolerance Network," accessed September 1, 2014, http://fedup.com.au.

88   Salicitic Sensitivity, accessed June 27, 2014, http://salicylatesensitivity.com.

89   Joan Breakey, "Are you Food Sensitive?" accessed September 1, 2014, http://www.foodintolerancepro.com.

90   Miguel A. Alvarez and M. V. Moreno-Arribas, "The Problem of Biogenic Amines in Fermented Foods and the Use of Potential Biogenic Amine-Degrading Microorganisms as a Solution," *Trends in Food Science & Technology* 39, no. 2 (2014) : 146–155; and S. Smolinska et al., "Histamine and Gut Mucosal Immune Regulation," *Allergy* 69, no. 3 (2014) : 273–281.

91   Smolinska, "Histamine and Gut," 273–281 (see note 90).

92   Ibid.

93   "The Failsafe Diet Explained," accessed September 1, 2014, http://www.failsafediet.com.

94   Joan Breakey, "Are you Food Sensitive?" accessed September 1, 2014, http://www.foodintolerancepro.com; Food Info, http://www.food-info.net/uk/qa/qa-fi27.htm; and The Australasian Society of Clinical Immunology and Allergy (ASCIA), www.allergy.org.au.

95   Joan Breakey, "Are you Food Sensitive?" http://www.foodintolerancepro.com; and "The Failsafe Diet

Explained," accessed September 1, 2014, http://www
.failsafediet.com.

96 Masood Sadiq Butt and M. Tauseef Sultan, "Coffee
and Its Consumption: Benefits and Risks," *Critical
Reviews in Food Science and Nutrition* 51, no. 4 (2011) :
363–373; and Neal D. Freedman et al., "Association
of Coffee Drinking with Total and Cause-Specific
Mortality," *New England Journal of Medicine* 366,
no. 20 (2012) : 1891–1904.

97 Nancy Clark, "Recognizing and Managing Exercise-
Associated Diarrhea," *ACSM's Health & Fitness Journal*
16, no. 3 (2012) : 22–26.

98 Wojciech Barg, Wojciech Medrala, and Anna
Wolanczyk-Medrala, "Exercise-Induced Anaphylaxis:
An Update on Diagnosis and Treatment," *Current
Allergy and Asthma Reports* 11, no. 1 (2011) : 45–51.

99 Stuart Carr et al., "CSACI Position Statement on
the Testing of Food-Specific IgG," *Allergy, Asthma, and
Clinical Immunology* 8, no. 1 (2012) : 12.

100 Ibid.

101 Fernando Fernández-Bañares, "Reliability of
Symptom Analysis During Carbohydrate Hydrogen-
Breath Tests," *Current Opinion in Clinical Nutrition
& Metabolic Care* 15, no. 5 (2012) : 494–498.

102 Shelley McGuire, "State Indicator Report on
Fruits and Vegetables, 2013, Centers for Disease
Control and Prevention," *Advances in Nutrition* 4,
no. 6 (2013) : 665–666; and Kirsten A. Grimm et al.,
"Household Income Disparities in Fruit and Vegetable
Consumption by State and Territory," *Journal of the
Academy of Nutrition and Dietetics* 112, no. 12 (2012) :
2014–2021.

103 N. Avena et al., "Further Developments in the
Neurobiology of Food and Addiction," *Nutrition* 28,
no. 4 (2012) : 341–343; and I. Koleva et al., "Alkaloids in
the Human Food Chain," *Molecular Nutrition & Food
Research* 56, no. 1 (2012) : 30–52; and J. Barrett and P.
Gibson, "Fermentable Oligosaccharides, Disaccharides,
Monosaccharides, and Polyols (FODMAPs) and
Nonallergic Food Intolerance," *Therapeutic Advances
in Gastroenterology* 5, no. 4 (2012) : 261–268.

104 Gary D. Foster et al., "Weight and Metabolic
Outcomes After 2 Years on a Low-Carbohydrate Versus
Low-Fat Diet," *Annals of Internal Medicine* 153, no. 3
(2010) : 147–157; and Jeffrey D. Browning et al., "Short-
Term Weight Loss and Hepatic Triglyceride Reduction,"
American Journal of Clinical Nutrition 93, no. 5 (2011) :
1048–1052.

105 Louise M. Burke et al., "Carbohydrates for Training
and Competition," *Journal of Sports Sciences* 29, suppl. 1
(2011) : S17–S27.

106 Naomi M. Cermak and Luc J. C. van Loon, "The Use
of Carbohydrates During Exercise as an Ergogenic Aid,"
Sports Medicine 43, no. 11 (2013) : 1139–1155.

107 John A. Hawley and Wee Kian Yeo, "Metabolic
Adaptations to a High-Fat Diet," in *The Encyclopaedia
of Sports Medicine*, vol. 19, ed. Ronald J. Maughan (Wiley
Online, 2014) : 166–173, doi 10.1002/9781118692318.

108 O. C. Witard et al., "High Dietary Protein Restores
Overreaching Induced Impairments in Leukocyte
Trafficking and Reduces the Incidence of Upper
Respiratory Tract Infection in Elite Cyclists," *Brain,
Behavior, and Immunity* 39 (July 2014) : 211–219.

109 Stuart M. Phillips and Luc J. C. van Loon, "Dietary
Protein for Athletes," *Journal of Sports Sciences* 29,
suppl. 1 (2011) : S29–S38.

110 Luc J. C. van Loon, "SSE #109 Is There a Need for
Protein Ingestion During Exercise?" http://www.gssi
web.org/Article/sse-109-is-there-a-need-for-protein
-ingestion-during-exercise.

111 Jane E. Kerstetter, Anne M. Kenny, and Karl L.
Insogna, "Dietary Protein and Skeletal Health: A Review
of Recent Human Research," *Current Opinion in
Lipidology* 22, no. 1 (2011) : 16–20.

112 M. Westerterp-Plantenga, S. Lemmens, and
K. Westerterp, "Dietary Protein: Its Role in Satiety,
Energetics, Weight Loss and Health," *British Journal
of Nutrition* 108, no. S2 (2012) : S105–S112; and R. Atallah
et al., "Long-Term Effects of 4 Popular Diets on Weight
Loss and Cardiovascular Risk Factors," *Circulation:
Cardiovascular Quality and Outcomes* 7, no. 6 (2014) :
815–827; and S. Pasiakos et al., "Whole-Body Protein

Turnover Response to Short-Term High-Protein Diets During Weight Loss," *International Journal of Obesity* 38, no. 7 (2014) : 1015–1018.

113 Elisa Couto Gomes, Albená Nunes Silva, and Marta Rubino de Oliveira, "Oxidants, Antioxidants, and the Beneficial Roles of Exercise-Induced Production of Reactive Species," *Oxidative Medicine and Cellular Longevity* (2012) .

114 Brandon W. Too et al., "Natural Versus Commercial Carbohydrate Supplementation and Endurance Running Performance," *Journal of International Society of Sports Nutrition* 9, no. 1 (2012) : 27.

115 Asker E. Jeukendrup, "Multiple Transportable Carbohydrates and Their Benefits," *Sports Science Exchange* 26, no. 108 (2013) : 1–5.

116 Ian Rollo et al., "Influence of Mouth Rinsing a Carbohydrate Solution on 1-H Running Performance," *Medicine and Science in Sports and Exercise* 42, no. 4 (2010) : 798–804; and Stephen C. Lane et al., "Effect of a Carbohydrate Mouth Rinse on Simulated Cycling Time-Trial Performance Commenced in a Fed or Fasted State," *Applied Physiology, Nutrition, and Metabolism* 38, no. 2 (2012) : 134–139.

INDEX

Note: Italic page numbers indicate photographs.

sugar, 12, 36, 38, 41 (table), 54; avoiding, 39; carbohydrates and, 90; eliminating, 37; inflammation and, 40; spotting, 40

sulfur, 47

supplements, 3, 48, 97; avoiding, 106

Sweet Potato Chocolate Chip Cookies, 188, *189*

Sweet Potato Hash Browns with Poached Eggs, 116, *117*

sweeteners: artificial, 40, 41 (table); avoiding, 39; eliminating, 37; listed, 39

symptoms, 17, 32, 74, 77, 83; food intolerance, 15 (table), 20, 24, 36, 73

syrups, listed, 39

tapioca flour, 79

10-Minute Mini-Carrot Cake, 184, *185*

thermogenic effect, 22

toxins, 11, 22, 50, 66

training, 4, 13, 36, 77, 95; adjustments in, 28; eating and, 28; energy and, 92; food intolerances and, 26, 27; intensity of, 89; nutrition and, 3; physical differences and, 27; recovery and, 88; stress fractures and, 3; weight gain and, 28–29

trans fats, 37, 41 (table); avoiding, 40

transglutaminase, 51

urinary system, 81; stress and, 21

USDA, unhealthy foods and, 37

vegan diet, 6, 47–48

vegans, 46

vegetables, 1, 2, 5, 37, 43, 47, 60, 62; carbohydrates and, 88, 89; chemicals in, 58; components of, 97; eating, 45, 50, 75; nutrient-dense, 56; pre-chopped, 107

vegetarian diet, 6, 47–48

vegetarians, 46, 47, 48

viruses, 10, 11, 53

vitamins, 10, 11, 28, 44, 46, 47, 48, 53, 54, 58, 97; absorbing, 92, 93; food intolerance and, 19; healthy, 45

vomiting, 14

walnuts, 45

Warm Shrimp, Pea, Shallot & Herb Salad, 140, *141*

weight gain, 12; carbohydrates and, 88; muscle mass and, 29; training and, 28–29

weight loss, 4, 6, 28–29; calorie-restricted, 97; protein and, 96, 97; sleep and, 29

wheat, 18, 20, 23, 30, 38, 88; derivatives, 49; inflammation and, 17

whey: eating, 53; protein powders, 53

Whole 30 program, described, 5

xylitol, 39

yeast, 18, 42 (table), 49

zinc, 32, 45, 46, 48

Zucchini Fritters, 126, *127*

ABOUT THE AUTHOR

Pip Taylor is an accredited practicing dietitian, sports dietitian, and professional triathlete. She holds a master's degree in nutrition and dietetics and postgraduate certifications in sports dietetics and sports nutrition.

As a professional triathlete, Pip has competed on the international circuit for the last 15 years, winning numerous major titles including ITU World Cup and Ironman 70.3 events and representing Australia on many occasions. As an athlete, Pip has experienced firsthand how small changes in nutrition can have a significant impact on health as well as on sports performance and recovery. Her passion for sports performance and interest in the human body ultimately led her to pursue a formal education in the field of nutrition. Global travel on the pro circuit—including time spent living in the United States and Europe—as well as exposure to and collaboration with other nutrition experts deepened her understanding of issues related to food, nutrition, and health and the unique requirements of each individual.

Pip's work as a dietitian has given her the opportunity to educate, engage, and entertain a wide variety of audiences on the value of eating real, whole foods. She consults with sports teams and individual clients, from professional athletes to corporate health programs and sports nutrition product developers. As a speaker and regular contributor to various magazines, web sites, and other media, Pip takes pride in her ability to entertain and engage, thus effectively encouraging athletes to achieve greater potential in their chosen sport and encouraging everyone to take steps toward better health and well-being.

When she is not out swimming, biking, or running around the beautiful North Coast of New South Wales, Australia, Pip can be found at the farmers market, in the kitchen, or cleaning up endless happy messes created by her two young children. Feeding her own family while also fueling for the demands of training has given Pip a real appreciation for the challenges associated with eating well on a daily basis. Born out of a genuine love of good food and the difference it makes, *The Athlete's Fix* is a guide to help others enjoy good food, better performance, and overall health.